You Will Get Through This

A MENTAL HEALTH FIRST-AID KIT

Help for
**DEPRESSION
ANXIETY
GRIEF**
and More

**JULIE RADICO, PsyD, ABPP
CHARITY O'REILLY, LPC
NICOLE HELVERSON, PsyD**

THE EXPERIMENT
NEW YORK

The Experiment, LLC
220 East 23rd Street, Suite 600
New York, NY 10010-4658
theexperimentpublishing.com

THE EXPERIMENT and its colophon are registered trademarks of The Experiment, LLC. Many of the designations used by manufacturers and sellers to distinguish their products are claimed as trademarks. Where those designations appear in this book and The Experiment was aware of a trademark claim, the designations have been capitalized.

The Experiment's books are available at special discounts when purchased in bulk for premiums and sales promotions as well as for fundraising or educational use. For details, contact us at info@theexperimentpublishing.com.

Library of Congress Cataloging-in-Publication Data

Names: Radico, Julie, author. | O'Reilly, Charity, author. | Helverson, Nicole, author.
Title: You will get through this : a mental health first-aid kit : help for depression, anxiety, grief, and more / Julie Radico, PsyD, ABPP, Charity O'Reilly, LPC, Nicole Helverson, PsyD.
Description: New York : The Experiment, [2024] | Includes bibliographical references and index.
Identifiers: LCCN 2024015080 (print) | LCCN 2024015081 (ebook) | ISBN 9781891011474 (trade paperback) | ISBN 9781891011481 (ebook)
Subjects: LCSH: Mental health--Popular works. | Mental health--United States--Popular works. | Mental health services--United States--Popular works. | Anxiety disorders--Treatment--Popular works. | Depression, Mental--Treatment--Popular works. | Neuroses--Treatment--Popular works.
Classification: LCC RA790 .R235 2024 (print) | LCC RA790 (ebook) | DDC 362.2--dc23/eng/20240501
LC record available at https://lccn.loc.gov/2024015080
LC ebook record available at https://lccn.loc.gov/2024015081

ISBN 978-1-891011-47-4
Ebook ISBN 978-1-891011-48-1

Cover design by Jack Dunnington
Text design and illustrations by Beth Bugler

Manufactured in the United States of America

First printing July 2024
10 9 8 7 6 5 4 3 2 1

To you, dear reader: May you find what you need within these pages.

CONTENTS

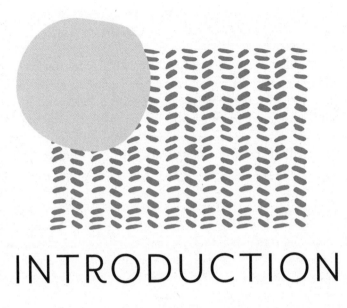

INTRODUCTION

I f you're reading this, you may know firsthand how hard it can be to find help when you're struggling with your mental health. Or maybe you've seen a loved one struggling and felt powerless. It can be challenging to reach out for support, especially if you have to call multiple clinicians or send several emails to get a response. It can be difficult to acknowledge when you need help, and yet it takes further strength and perseverance to actually get it.

With that in mind, we've framed this book using the biopsychosocial model—a psychological model in which you are viewed as a whole person. This is not always common in the US health care system, which is segmented based on specialty, where you see one clinician for your foot and another for your throat. In considering the whole of you, we discuss the biological (physical), psychological (mental and emotional), and social (relationships, finances, culture) factors that may impact your healing journey.

The Challenges of Being Human

Being human, you have likely faced challenges with your physical, mental, and social health. Considering how closely tied all facets of our health are, there's often a ripple effect that occurs when one area is out of balance. For instance, if you're struggling with your mood (psychological), you may find your relationships are suffering because you don't have energy to sustain them (social). If you're getting to work late or missing days because of your low mood and energy (psychological/biological), your finances may be impacted (social). Your limited finances may prevent you from seeking the care you need or paying your bills (social), which places further strain on your mood and well-being (psychological/biological). These interlinking challenges highlight the importance of the biopsychosocial model. As mental health clinicians, we understand that your mental and social health are important components of your overall heath, and we've written this book with the whole you in mind.

The Limitations of the Mental Health System

The current mental health system has many shortcomings, and yet being able to navigate this system is often the key to finding the support you need. Diagnosis is usually necessary for insurance to cover treatment, yet the manual used to diagnose that we cite in this book, the *Diagnostic and Statistical Manual of Mental Disorders* (DSM), has long been criticized for upholding racism, ableism, and a lack of understanding of neurodiversity.[1] This limiting view of the diversity of humankind does not uphold the health and well-being of every individual. Efforts have been made in recent years to address these biases, although we are not yet where we need to be.

We know the importance of being connected with supports who approach care in a holistic, multicultural, and trauma-informed way and with whom you feel safe, seen, and truly supported. You are unique, and your journey through mental health challenges should be, too. For example, a diagnosis may feel like a label to you, and therefore you may experience it as limiting or harmful. Or the opposite may be true; a diagnosis may provide the opportunity and empowerment you need to find healing, whether on your own or in treatment. Decisions about your mental health care are highly personal. In this book, we provide many options for you to consider, as we try to give you the information you may need to navigate your way through the existing system.

Please note: This book is not a replacement for professional mental health care, and through authoring this book we are not acting in the role as your mental health professional. We encourage you to speak with a health professional about what you read here and how it can be applied to you. We hope this book will help you understand and manage the ups and downs or perhaps it will help you have a conversation with a loved one who has been struggling. No matter the reason you picked up this book, we are so glad you did.

There is a lot of information (and misinformation) out there when it comes to what works for our mental health. We used the current research as our guide; however, we need to acknowledge that even the world of scientific research is biased.[2] Research studies historically overrepresent white, college-educated, middle-class people, which is not fully representative of our world. Even in studies as recent as the writing of this book more than 75 percent of participants were white,[3] and most of the people conducting research are also white and predominantly male.[4] As a result, there are many gaps in the research, especially if you are not a white, straight, cisgendered person. It's also important for us to address our own privilege of having access to education and training, as well as living in white, cisgendered, able bodies. We recognize our limitations and have made efforts to be mindful of diversity, equity, inclusion, and accessibility factors throughout this book. By using our combined fifty years of experience as therapists, we hope to fill the gaps in the imbalanced research with practical, therapy-tested techniques you can try at home, or to guide you to find professional help if and when it is needed.

How to Use This Book

This book is divided into five parts.

- Mental Health explores common disorders such as anxiety and depression.
- Social Health covers the many ways relationships impact our functioning.
- Sexual Health discusses the psychological impacts of experiences such as sexual assault and intimate partner violence.

- Physical Health explores how bodily factors like poor sleep can impact mental well-being.

- Getting Support provides guidance for getting the support you need, whether you need help navigating insurance or breaking up with your therapist.

Each chapter is broken down into sections for easy navigation. First, a chapter introduction provides background. Then we identify a variety of professional treatment approaches that you may consider as well as practical coping skills you can use right away. Next, each chapter covers barriers to receiving help and other challenges specific to the issue. It provides guidance on how to start conversations and give support whether you are the one struggling or a loved one is. Finally, we provide an example of what coping with a particular struggle can look like in real life and suggest additional resources that may be of help. Many chapters also include sidebars that detail what the latest research says about how common the struggle is, how it impacts your brain and body, and other mental and physical health concerns that often accompany the issue. And because we know that children and adolescents all too often struggle with their mental health, we include icons next to tips that are especially helpful when the person is a child. For help with unfamiliar mental health terms, check out the glossary at the end of the book.

Please be mindful of your limits and boundaries while reading this book. Give yourself permission to take breaks, or even skip over a section if you're finding it stressful. Part of the healing process is learning when to give yourself space and when to challenge yourself. This book does not need to be read in any particular order or within any time frame. You get to decide what this healing process looks like for you. You can read this book from front to back, or just read the chapters that speak to you.

While certain chapters may resonate with you now, you may also find this book to be a helpful tool in the future, as your needs change over time. We hope you'll consider this book to be a lifelong companion that will be there for you whenever you need it.

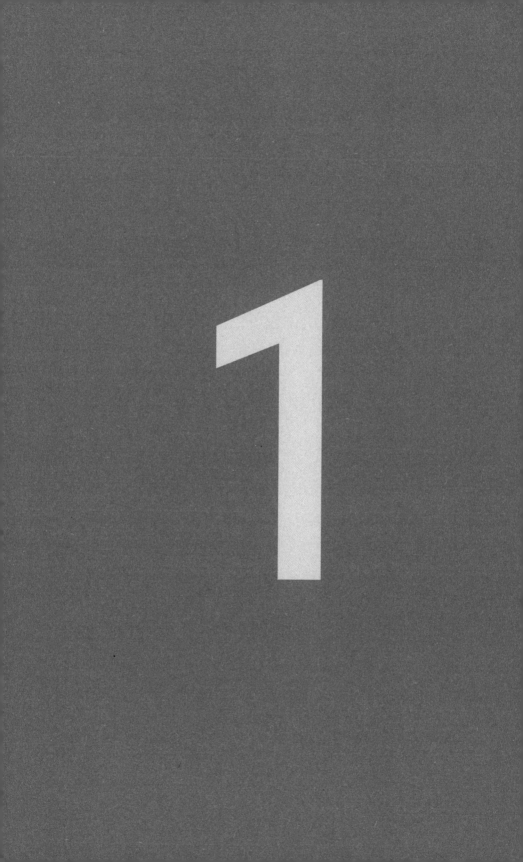

MENTAL
HEALTH

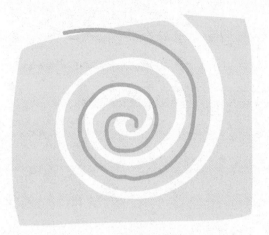

1

DEPRESSION

I f you have suffered from depression, you know just how debilitating it can be. Depression can make you feel as though it's impossible to do the tasks life requires of you, and it can even make you wonder if life is still worth living at all.

Feeling sad, angry, overwhelmed, or helpless because terrible things are happening to or around you is completely normal. However, there may be a time when you feel overcome with those emotions and unable to cope. Under these circumstances, you may have an adjustment disorder, which is diagnosed within three months of experiencing a stressor that causes anxiety, depressed mood, or disturbance of emotions and conduct (such as lying or physical aggression), or combinations of these conditions. The depressed mood that you may experience due to an adjustment disorder is different from experiencing depression. Depression is a low mood that lasts weeks, months, or years, with ripple effects in other areas of your health, such as your sleep, energy levels, and appetite. Treating depression can help you feel better prepared to face the realities of the world around you.

There are many types of depression. Throughout this chapter, we'll be focusing on Major Depressive Disorder. To be diagnosed with Major Depressive Disorder, you need to display at least five of the following nine symptoms for at least two weeks.[1]

- Depressed mood (feeling sad, empty, or hopeless) lasting almost all day, nearly every day. (In children and adolescents, this can present itself as an irritable mood.)

- Markedly diminished interest or pleasure in all, or almost all, activities lasting almost all day, nearly every day.

- Significant unintentional change in weight, or a significant decrease or increase in appetite nearly every day. (In children, this can present itself as failure to make expected weight gains.)

- Insomnia (difficulty falling asleep or staying asleep) or hypersomnia (sleeping longer than usual) nearly every day.

- Psychomotor changes (movements being more fidgety and agitated or being more sluggish) severe enough to be observable by others.

- Tiredness, fatigue, low energy, or decreased efficiency with routine tasks nearly every day.

- Feelings of worthlessness or excessive, inappropriate, or delusional guilt nearly every day.

- Diminished ability to think, concentrate, or make decisions nearly every day.

- Recurrent thoughts of death (not just fear of dying), suicidal ideation without a specific plan, or a suicide attempt or a specific plan for dying by suicide.

As you can see, depression can look different for each person. You may have an increased appetite, find you are sleeping more, and feel generally slower, while someone else might have a decreased appetite, trouble sleeping, and feel irritable. You may also experience only a single bout of depression or have recurrent episodes.

Of note, if you are experiencing depression, you may also have mood episodes in which you feel almost the opposite of depressed, even feeling better than back to normal. You may feel energized without the need to sleep, may make risky decisions that get you or your family into trouble, and may be more talkative or argumentative than usual. You may have periods lasting at least four to seven days in a row in which you experience such hypomanic or manic symptoms. This means that instead of being diagnosed with Major Depressive Disorder (depression) you may instead meet criteria for Bipolar Disorder. Our focus here is depression, but this is important to consider when you are experiencing depression as the medications are different from those used to treat Bipolar Disorder.

There are many types of depression not addressed in this book that will be important for you to discuss with your health care clinician. Since depression can show up in numerous unique ways, the best coping strategies for you or your loved one will depend on how your particular case manifests.

What Professional Help May Look Like

Treatment for depression depends on how severe the symptoms are. For mild depression, low-intensity interventions such as therapy and self-help guides can be beneficial. Exercise can also help prevent and manage symptoms.[2]

MEDICATION

For moderate to severe depression, medication or a combination of medication and therapy are helpful in its treatment.[3] Since antidepressants (for example, selective serotonin reuptake inhibitors, SSRIs) come with potential side effects, it's important to talk to your medical clinician about which may work best for you. Your clinician may start you on medications alone, since they are often easier to access than therapy.

If your depression persists despite therapy and medication, ketamine treatment[4] may be helpful. Such treatment should always be done under the supervision of a medical or mental health professional.

Talking with your medical clinician about depression can be overwhelming, so before meeting with them, write down any concerns and questions you have and bring that list with you to your appointment. During the appointment, take notes to reference afterward.

COGNITIVE BEHAVIORAL THERAPY

Cognitive Behavioral Therapy (CBT) is the psychological intervention with the most evidence for helping depression, but Problem-Solving Therapy (PST) and Interpersonal Therapy are also helpful.[5] CBT can be effectively delivered to treat depression in different settings. For mild to moderate depression, it is effective in the primary care setting and a good first step if you are seeking treatment.[6] CBT provided through a computer program is also helpful for mild depression.[7] Several components of CBT, including cognitive restructuring, behavioral activation, and homework assignments, have been found to be the most helpful.[8]

PROBLEM-SOLVING THERAPY

Developed from CBT, PST helps you take a step-by-step approach to problem solving in an effort to reduce your depression. These steps can include defining the problem, setting realistic goals, brainstorming possible solutions, choosing the best approach, and carrying it out to see if it works or not.[9]

THE RESEARCH SAYS . . .

You Are Not Alone

Around the world, 322 million people are living with depression.[12] It is more common in women than men and affects people of all ages. Depression is one of the leading causes of disability and accounts for 2.72 million years of life lost due to ill-health, disability, or early death in people in just the United States alone.[13] Due to how common depression is, you have likely experienced depression or know others who have.

In a 2019 census bureau sample, 6.6 percent of the general population was estimated to be experiencing depression.[14] In comparison, a sample from April 2020 during the COVID-19 pandemic, found that 23.5 percent of respondents were likely to screen positive for depression. This finding points to how feelings of depression can be affected by external circumstances.

INTERPERSONAL THERAPY

Interpersonal Therapy is a short-term therapy that focuses on your past and current relationship patterns. Your treatment may focus on a person important to you that died, a struggle with a partner, or another important life change.[10] All of these stressors potentially contribute to the depression you experience.

ATTACHMENT-BASED FAMILY THERAPY

Attachment-Based Family Therapy (ABFT) is an evidence-based (researched) treatment for adolescents experiencing depression.[11] ABFT involves both the child and their caregivers to promote healthy attachment. (You can learn more about attachment in chapters 7 and 10.) An important principle is that kids need to heal in the context of their closest relationships. When we put a child or teen in the role of "identified patient," and separate them from the group, they cannot receive the secure attachment and modeling they need to recover. As hard as it can be to have the time or energy, inviting the whole family into healing is a crucial part of your child or teen's wellness.

Strategies to Try

If your depression symptoms are "subclinical" (not reaching the diagnostic criteria, although still difficult to experience), you may benefit from self-help strategies. In particular, research suggests that exercise,[15] light therapy,[16] and maintaining a daily routine[17] may help prevent or decrease subclinical depression, while social isolation tends to make it worse.[18] These strategies may also be helpful if you are diagnosed with depression, though will likely not be enough to improve your depression on their own. So, while regular exercise, keeping up with healthy routines like getting out in sunlight every day, and being around loved ones may not effectively treat clinical depression, they may prevent it from worsening.

PRACTICE REFRAMING YOUR THOUGHTS

Cognitive Restructuring means recognizing your automatic thoughts and cognitive distortions (unhelpful thinking habits) and reframing them to develop different points of view about situations.[19]

Automatic thoughts are those you have throughout the day. They pop into your head, seemingly without prompting. Your automatic thoughts are often affected by your past experiences. Examples of unhelpful automatic thoughts include *I'm a failure*, and *This will never get better*.

To reframe these thoughts, first recognize that thoughts are not facts. Next, practice reframing them by identifying one that is more fair and realistic. One way of doing this is to ask yourself *What would I say to a loved one if I heard them say to themselves what I just thought?*

> **THE RESEARCH SAYS . . .**
>
> **This Is How Depression Impacts Your Brain and Body**
>
> It's likely that many regions of the brain are involved in depression, including areas related to emotions (the amygdala), regulating our bodies (the thalamus), decision making (the striatum), memory (the hippocampus), and thinking (the prefrontal and cingulate cortex).[20]

SING A SONG

Help children reframe their thoughts by turning the new positive thoughts into a song. Have them pick their favorite song, and then put new words (the positive thoughts) to the music. This makes the positive thoughts both fun and easy to remember. (This tip works for grown-ups, too!)

USE BEHAVIORAL ACTIVATION

Behavioral Activation is a strategy that aims to increase your awareness of your emotions, engage in repeated practice, and give you opportunities for learning through your experiences.[21] Basically, it helps you recognize when you have stopped engaging in healthy or enjoyable behaviors due to feeling depressed. The goal is to start increasing your activity levels, which can have a positive effect on your mood. Behavioral Activation can include self-monitoring, activity scheduling, reducing avoidance, and replacing avoidance strategies with valued alternative actions.[22]

Self-monitoring and activity scheduling include observing your mood along with your daily activities to see their connection. This includes tracking your behaviors in a log that can include things like what led to a behavior, what the behavior was, how long you engaged in the behavior, and how you felt throughout.[23] This information helps you develop a plan to increase the number of pleasant activities and positive interactions with your environment.

Practicing such strategies on your own is helpful, and we encourage you to try them. However, it may not replace the benefit of therapy. It has been found that the more human support (time with a coach or therapist) integrated into CBT has a positive connection with the success of the interventions.[24]

Barriers to Feeling Better

THE DEMOTIVATIONAL EFFECTS OF DEPRESSION

Depression can destroy motivation, causing you to feel stuck. The symptoms of depression create obstacles to engaging consistently in the evidence-based treatments that could help relieve those symptoms. It can cause us to feel simultaneously low in energy, disinterested, and hopeless, thereby making it hard to take the steps to find a therapist and actively engage in therapy, or to participate in a healthy routine at home.

Some of our clients have compared the process of healing from depression to having a broken leg and being asked to walk in order to heal. The lack of motivation and energy can make it feel impossible to take the steps needed to recover. If this sounds like you, medication may be an important support in your recovery.

If your depression makes even having the energy or motivation to take your medication regularly feel impossible, ask your clinician about the possibility of switching to an injectable medication. It's also okay to ask a loved one to help you remember to take your medication.

NEGATIVE THINKING FEEDBACK LOOPS

Negative thinking, especially when filled with cognitive distortions, can keep you feeling unmotivated and hopeless. If your thoughts discourage you from trying or make you think things will never get better, they will keep you stuck on a self-fulfilling prophecy. Feelings of shame and guilt about struggling to break out of your depression serve only to make it tougher to improve your mood.

Minimizing your struggles can be a barrier in recognizing that you are experiencing depression. See if you can try and "befriend" your depression instead. This doesn't mean you have to like your depression, but instead try to make space for it, like you would a friend (maybe just not your best friend!). You may find that when you befriend it, you have more energy because you were using so much of it to fight its existence.

THE RESEARCH SAYS . . .

You May Also Experience These Things

If you have depression, you are more likely to also experience Persistent Depressive Disorder (depressed mood most days for at least two years), Obsessive-Compulsive Disorder, Post-Traumatic Stress Disorder (page 57), Alcohol Use Disorder (page 189), Psychotic Disorder, Antisocial Personality Disorder, eating disorders (page 177), and anxiety disorders (page 19), such as Generalized Anxiety Disorder (page 31), Panic Disorder (page 48), Agoraphobia, and Social Anxiety Disorder (page 40).[25]

GIVE YOUR DEPRESSION A NAME

A child may like the idea of "naming" their depression in order to befriend it. For example, they may call their depression "Sad Sammy" as a way to refer to its visits, and to have a way to ask their depression what it needs and how it can be helped.

This also helps children externalize the experience of depression, so they know it's not the core of who they are, even though it can feel that way sometimes. Like most strategies for kids, it may help you, too.

How to Communicate About Depression

IF YOU'RE THE ONE DEALING WITH DEPRESSION

It's important not to isolate yourself from others but to let them know how they can best support you. Unless you tell them, others can only guess. Expressing what you feel will be the most helpful. Say things like, "I need some space right now," "Can you just sit with me and keep me company?" or "I would like to feel included."

Give yourself permission to ask for help with basic life tasks. You could say, "I need help with cleaning my home, because I know I can't do it on my own right now, yet the dirty house is making me feel even worse," or "Could you come with me grocery shopping, because I know I can't do it on my own right now?" This applies to asking for support or companionship when attending your medical appointments, too.

It's important to be open about your safety. Ask others to check in on you and to implement your crisis plan if needed. (Find information about creating a crisis plan on page 228.)

IF A LOVED ONE IS DEALING WITH DEPRESSION

Respect the limits they set while also taking actions to demonstrate your care with their permission. This can look like making them a meal or watching a movie together at home. Even if they have not expressed suicidal thoughts, as these are common in those with depression, it is helpful to have open conversations about safety and suicide, offer to call 988 or take them to the emergency room, and call on additional support from trusted family members and friends. Tell them you're there to listen or sit with them while they call 988 or their therapist. Make efforts to be nonjudgmental, and don't blame or shame your loved one or yourself in these conversations. Most importantly, just be present.

IF THE PERSON DEALING WITH DEPRESSION IS A CHILD

Do not ever take mental health symptoms lightly just because it is happening to a child. Suicide is the second leading cause of death for US children aged ten to fourteen.[26]

Children use the language of play. You can help your child find ways to express their feelings about their depression by using art, music, dance, puppets, and other types of play. Above all, take them and their feelings seriously.

What Coping with Depression Can Look Like in Real Life

Over the past several months, Carl has started to notice changes in his mood. He's found it harder to get out of bed and others have commented on how he seems less energetic and tends to do things more slowly. Carl finds himself canceling plans because he feels so tired all the time. He has lost interest in his hobbies and started to feel hopeless.

Carl seeks help by scheduling an appointment with his primary care clinician. They say he may be experiencing a major depressive episode. Since he had similar symptoms a few years ago, they tell him that it sounds like he may be having "recurrent episodes." Carl shares that he's had some thoughts about death. He expresses that sometimes he wishes he could go to sleep and not wake up (passive suicidal ideation). He doesn't have thoughts about hurting or killing himself, so he and his clinician discuss the Suicide and Crisis Lifeline (988) and how he can call or text that number for 24-7 support. The national line routes to Carl's local crisis center, so he would talk to someone who knows the specific resources in his area.

Since Carl's depression symptoms are in the severe range, they discuss how both therapy and medication can be considered for treatment. Carl is willing to try both, so he's started on a low dose of an antidepressant called an SSRI, a selective serotonin reuptake inhibitor. The medication is supposed to help affect the serotonin in Carl's brain to improve his depression, though it may take four to six weeks, or even up to twelve weeks, to feel the effects.

Carl starts seeing a therapist who teaches him about Cognitive Behavioral Therapy. He begins by adding one enjoyable hobby back into his daily activities. He also catches and examines his negative thoughts and recognizes the distortions that come up. He finds that he assumes bad things will happen (*I'm going to fail*) and judges himself with "should" statements (*I should feel better already*). He practices reframing these thoughts as *Telling myself I am going to fail is not helpful. Instead, I can ask for support if the task feels too big*, and *I need to give myself time to heal and create healthier coping strategies*.

Carl also focuses on developing a routine he'll actually stick to. He tries to go for a walk every day, and to see at least one friend a week. Over time, although his depressive symptoms have not gone away altogether, he does see an improvement.

If you are feeling suicidal: Depression can be accompanied by thoughts of death or even plans of suicide. Such thoughts are common and are important to talk about with others. If you are feeling suicidal, call or text 988 or go to your local emergency room. Additional resources can be found in the Resources that follow.

READING LIST AND OTHER RESOURCES

It is important to seek help during these times, to get the support to help ride out the intensity of those thoughts. Here are some important numbers.

National Suicide and Crisis Lifeline: Call or text 988

BlackLine (a crisis call line that prioritizes BIPOC): Call or text 800-604-5841

Trans Lifeline: Call 877-565-8860

NAMI HelpLine provides information, referrals, and guidance to anyone living with mental health conditions as well as their families and caregivers, clinicians, and other members of the public: Call 800-950-NAMI (6264) Monday through Friday, 10:00 AM to 10:00 PM EST, or send an email to helpline@nami.org.

SAMHSA's National Helpline is available 24-7, 365 days a year, for free, confidential treatment referrals and information. The service helps individuals and families struggling with mental and/or substance use disorders and help is available in English and Spanish: 1-800-662-HELP (4357).

The Feeling Good Handbook: The Groundbreaking Program with Powerful New Techniques and Step-by-Step Exercises to Overcome Depression, Conquer Anxiety, and Enjoy Greater Intimacy by David D. Burns provides specific strategies to help your communication and building your self-esteem.

How to Keep House While Drowning: A Gentle Approach to Cleaning and Organizing by K. C. Davis may help you get back on your feet when depression leaves you feeling too overwhelmed to do basic life tasks.

Peace Is a Practice: An Invitation to Breathe Deep and Find a New Rhythm for Life by Morgan Harper Nichols explores many ways to "practice peace" that can be helpful for depression, anxiety, and more.

The Hilarious World of Depression is a podcast that aims to normalize your experiences with depression while also providing coping strategies and sometimes even laughter.

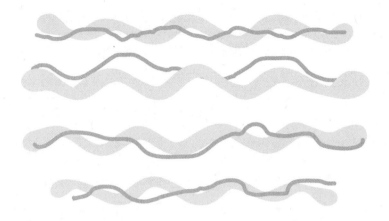

2

ANXIETY

I f you are experiencing anxiety, you are not alone. It's estimated that 264 million people around the world are living with anxiety disorders.[1] We will explore subclinical anxiety, meaning the symptoms you are experiencing may negatively impact your life but do not meet criteria for a diagnosis such as Generalized Anxiety Disorder, Panic Disorder, or Social Anxiety Disorder. We'll discuss these disorders, which can lead to significant disruptions in functioning and quality of life, in other chapters.

Common symptoms of anxiety are feeling restless or on edge, having trouble concentrating, feeling irritable, having racing thoughts, and feeling unable to relax.[2] You may feel some anxiety leading up to a new activity or a difficult conversation with a loved one. This is a normal part of the human experience, not a "disorder," as uncomfortable as it may be at times.

Anxiety can manifest physically as well as mentally. You may experience a racing heartbeat, shortness of breath, dizziness, or nausea, along with other symptoms. Some people may clench their jaw or pick at their fingernails or experience relentless negative thoughts, also called rumination. Regardless of how it may present, it's helpful to know what contributes to the anxiety you feel, and what will help you manage it effectively.

There are two main types of anxiety: State Anxiety and Trait Anxiety. State Anxiety is when you quickly respond to something that feels threatening to your safety. Trait Anxiety is long-term anxiety that sticks with you continuously and can be considered part of your personality.[3] You may get stuck with anxious thoughts because, as a child, you didn't learn another way to cope with your anxiety. Therefore, as an adult, when you experience anxious thoughts, you may not always realize that you have options at your disposal other than just rumination.

In this chapter, we will look specifically at the dynamic between perfectionism and anxiety. In perfectionism, you place unrealistic standards on yourself (such as to never make a mistake) and often engage in damaging, self-critical talk (for example, "I'm never enough"). Perfectionism is a risk factor for anxiety, as well as for eating disorders and depression.[4]

The likelihood of experiencing perfectionism has steadily increased over the years.[5] Comparing yourself negatively to others, such as through social media, can contribute to feelings of depression, anxiety, and feeling like you need to be perfect. We hope you find some helpful tools in this chapter to assist you or your loved one to better cope with anxiety and decrease the need for perfectionism.

What Professional Help May Look Like

COGNITIVE BEHAVIORAL THERAPY

You may find Cognitive Behavioral Therapy (CBT) helpful in managing and reducing anxiety and perfectionism.[6] CBT helps you to identify your thoughts, feelings, and behaviors, how they impact you, and those that help you feel empowered.[11]

Your CBT therapist may also teach you mindfulness techniques. Mindfulness has been shown to assist with many of the symptoms of and factors that cause anxiety, including the workplace stress and burnout that contribute to the anxiety of many adults today.[12] (For more on work stress and burnout, see chapter 12.)

SOMATIC THERAPIES

Somatic (body-based) therapies such as Neurofeedback, Sensorimotor Therapy, and Somatic Experiencing are also useful for treating anxiety in a therapy setting.[13] We will now look at somatic options you can try at home.

Strategies to Try

NOTICE HOW YOUR BODY FEELS

Your body and brain are interconnected in everything you do, including how you experience anxiety. See if you can notice where anxiety is revealing itself in your body. It may be in your chest or stomach, although it could be anywhere. If it's comfortable, gently place a hand on that part of your body and experience being with the sensation. Notice how the sensation isn't trying to hurt you, it's just communicating something. You can direct gentle breath to that part of your body, or talk to it. For example, you could say, "I see you, anxiety, and I appreciate how you are trying to notify me

---

THE RESEARCH SAYS . . .

This Is How Anxiety Impacts Your Brain and Body

Several areas of your brain are active when you experience anxiety, including those connected to your emotions (the amygdala), feelings of stability related to changes in hunger and blood pressure (the thalamus), and your thoughts (the prefrontal cortex).[14]

Scientists are working on identifying the relationship between stress and anxiety in our brains, with a likely strong two-way connection between the stress we experience and more significant anxiety, whether or not you have been diagnosed with an anxiety disorder.[15]

that something could be wrong. I don't see anything wrong right now, so let's just take a few breaths." Once your body feels more relaxed, you'll have moved out of the anxiety response, and be in a place of greater clarity to try one of the next strategies.

MOVEMENT

Releasing anxiety from your body, also known as "discharge," is another important step. Discharge can be as varied as taking a walk, going for a run, jumping on a mini trampoline, or having a solo dance party. You can also vigorously shake out your limbs.

PRACTICE MINDFULNESS

Mindfulness is the act of paying attention to the present moment without judgment.[16] While this is easy to say, it can be difficult to practice.

Choose a daily short period of time to be mindful, such as when you are brushing your teeth. What do you usually think about when you brush your teeth? You may think about the day ahead, or the worrisome things from the day that just passed. While practicing mindfulness, you instead notice exactly what is happening as you brush your teeth, such as the taste of the toothpaste. And instead of judging what you notice as good or bad, you simply accept what is. After a few moments, you have successfully practiced mindfulness! Building on this each day strengthens this important muscle for managing anxiety. It's important to note that if your thoughts drift away, that's okay! Just pull them back to the present moment.

BREATHE

Mindful breathing can be effective in bringing balance and calm to your body and mind.[17] By using breath to focus on the body, you are tricking your brain into thinking you are calm, which allows it to slow its racing thoughts. If you are breathing slowly and deeply and the muscles of your body are relaxed, your brain has a hard time thinking you are in danger and is therefore more willing to let go of your anxiety.

Nasal breathing: Count slowly to 4 as you inhale through your nose, pause for a moment, then breathe out to a count of 8 (the exhale should be longer than the inhale, which prompts the nervous system to begin to calm). Counting the length of each breath can be helpful in managing rumination and overthinking. To start, try a cycle of 4 inhales and exhales.

Another option is to add a mantra or positive statement to your intentional breathing, which can help to focus your mind and relax your body. For example, on an inhale, say to yourself "I breathe in relaxation"; on the exhale, say "I breathe out stress."

"Voo" breathing: Slowly breathe in through your nose. On the exhale, slowly release the word "voo"—it should sound more like "voooooooooooo" and is sometimes called the "foghorn breath" because it sounds like a foghorn when done correctly. This breath has the benefit of toning the vagus nerve, which is the longest cranial nerve that humans have, going from the brain to the gut. It's responsible for your stress and inflammatory responses.[18] If you think about where you feel most of your anxiety in your body, you'll probably notice it's somewhere along that nerve—whether in your throat, chest, or belly.

Cookie breathing: Ask the child to imagine a tray of warm cookies in front of them (or another food they like), and then to breathe in slowly through their nose, imagining that they are inhaling the scent of the cookies. Then, they will *slowwwwly* breathe out through their mouths, to cool the cookies down. This helps people of all ages to appreciate and embody the slow exhale that is needed for breathing techniques.

CARRY A COMFORT ITEM
Some kids like having a worry rock they can carry in their pocket, and when they feel nervous they can squeeze their feelings into the rock. Others like a worry jar or a worry journal to use before school or bed, where they can contain their worries.

GATHER EVIDENCE FOR AND AGAINST YOUR ANXIETY
A great CBT homework assignment is for you to gather the evidence for and against what you are anxious about. For example, if you are anxious because you didn't do something perfectly, what is the evidence that it's true? That may be easy for you to think about, but make sure it's concrete evidence, not just thoughts in your head. Next, try to collect evidence against that anxious thought. You can ask others, review past experiences, or play the imagined script through to the end, where you may find that the feared outcome isn't quite as bad as your anxiety made it seem.

FOCUS ON THE POSITIVE

When you're anxious, it can be challenging to recognize the positives. Make efforts to consciously think about positive experiences you have each day. It can be as simple as enjoying a cup of coffee to having a meaningful interaction with a dear friend. Write it down as a means of "collecting the data" to show you that there are positive experiences happening in your world.

KID-FRIENDLY TIP If you're helping a child track their positive experiences, it can help to use visual aids, such as daily stickers or drawing a picture that represents the positive experience.

Looking for the positives shouldn't be confused with toxic positivity, which involves thinking only about the positives while ignoring important difficulties. (For more on this, see page 103.)

PUT A LABEL ON NEGATIVE THOUGHTS

If the anxious thoughts persist, try pulling up a list of common cognitive distortions on the internet (they have names such as "catastrophizing," "mind reading," or "fortune telling") and see what resonates. Sometimes seeing that there's a name for the way you are thinking can be illuminating.

STICK TO A REGULAR ROUTINE

A healthy morning routine may put you in a better mindset at the onset of your day. This is particularly helpful if you experience anxiety in the morning, often caused by activities such as caretaking for family members or watching the news. A better routine may look like avoiding using your phone until after breakfast (this includes not checking your work emails), taking a moment to stretch, visualizing your day going well, or doing something you enjoy. The intention is to decrease anxiety-inducing activities in the morning and engage in soothing activities so you feel you have more emotional resources to start your day.

JOURNAL

Setting aside time each night, each week, or whenever you feel inspired to explore your thoughts and expectations can be helpful in uncovering where you may benefit from a shift in perspective. The following are some self-reflection prompts to get you started.

- What are my expectations of myself? Do I think they are truly fair?

- Would I expect that of anyone else?

- Are these expectations impacting my physical, social, or mental health in any way?
- Do I feel as though I have an identity outside of work/caretaking/etc.?
- How have I defined my value?
- How do I know when I've reached perfection? Do I know what I consider perfect? Do I actually believe anyone can be perfect?
- How does anxiety feel for me? Where do I feel it in my body?
- If my anxiety could speak, what would it be saying to me?
- What need is my anxiety trying to help me meet?
- What kind words do I want to say to my anxiety?

PRACTICE SELF-COMPASSION

Learning to give yourself grace and compassion is critical when it comes to changing negative self-talk (for example, "I am never good enough").[19]

Consider changing your self-talk to include *I am learning to be kind to myself*, and *It's okay for me to be kind to myself*. Since reducing anxiety can also improve your physical health, consider phrases such as *Taking time to rest helps keep me healthy*; *I don't have to earn rest*; and *I'm investing in my health by reducing my stress*. Every time you think kinder thoughts, you are reinforcing new thought patterns in your brain and coming to believe that you are worth your own loving time and effort.[20]

Know that it may take time before the message sinks in and becomes a reality; being kind to ourselves can be a long journey. To help yourself make consistent progress, try setting aside a specific regular time to practice these thoughts, like whenever you log into social media or wash your hands.

Barriers to Feeling Better

POSITIVE OUTCOMES FROM ANXIETY

Perfectionism and anxiety can be rewarding, as they may drive you to push yourself harder and achieve more. This creates an unhealthy feedback loop that is hard, although not impossible, to break.

For example, you may use procrastination as a way to wait until your anxiety is at a high so that it "motivates" you to succeed. Using anxiety against yourself in this way is not healthy. Perhaps befriending your anxiety would be a better approach. If you use "parts work" techniques (such as Internal Family Systems Therapy, where you are encouraged to look at your emotions as though they are separate subpersonalities or aspects of your whole self),[21] you will reframe this by saying, "Thank you to the part of myself who pushed me to perform and achieve through college and to get my first job. I appreciate how far you got me. However, now I'd like to just relax and enjoy how far you helped me reach!"

LACK OF SLEEP

Anxiety often makes it hard to get restful sleep, and poor sleep can lead to more anxiety. Sleep troubles are a common symptom and can also be a by-product of perfectionism.[22] When we aren't rested, it's harder for us to relax. (For more on sleep, see chapter 21.)

TOXIC OR DEMANDING ENVIRONMENTS

Our surroundings can be a huge contributor to our health. Reflect on how you feel in each of your environments, such as work, your relationship, religion, home, and so on. Are they healthy? Making too many demands? Do you feel allowed to be yourself? It can be challenging to manage anxiety effectively in toxic and/or demanding environments. It puts our minds and bodies in a near constant fight, flight, freeze, or fawn (people-pleasing, placating) response. (See chapter 10 for help setting boundaries in unhealthy environments.)

BEING OVERWORKED

Rarely taking time off is a major barrier to managing the anxiety and perfectionism you may experience. By not taking a break, you don't get a chance to rest and restore. It's okay to take care of yourself! Prioritize scheduling breaks lasting at least ten minutes throughout the day, and give yourself a weekly break of at least several hours. Such breaks may help you be more productive overall.

MINDLESSLY "CHECKING OUT"

Mindlessly scrolling on your phone is probably doing you more harm than good. Overexposure to the twenty-four-hour news cycle creates additional anxiety and can activate your nervous system in unhealthy ways.

Try setting limits on your phone time, including leaving your phone outside the bedroom while you sleep and putting it on airplane mode when you relax or during that time off we encouraged you to take.

How to Communicate About Anxiety

IF YOU'RE THE ONE EXPERIENCING ANXIETY

Speak openly about your boundaries. This may mean asking others to help you keep those boundaries. You may say, "I am working on focusing more on myself and obsessing less about work. If you notice that I am canceling plans with you, please gently point that out to me."

At work, this may involve saying, "I am available during the hours of 9 AM to 5 PM during the workweek and will not be responding to emails or phone calls before or after those hours." Then, hold firm to that boundary!

IF A LOVED ONE IS EXPERIENCING ANXIETY

Here are a few questions to ask.

- Do you need me to just listen or are you looking for solutions? Or a combination of both?

- What is it like for you to live with this anxiety?

- How can I best support you?

- Do you need a ride to your appointment? Do you want me to come with you?

These questions help you take a curious and nonjudgmental stance in which you let the person tell you how you can best support them. You will want to avoid pushing the person out of their comfort zone or shaming them by comparing them to others. It is important to honor their pace in challenging their anxiety or in setting boundaries.

IF THE PERSON EXPERIENCING ANXIETY IS A CHILD

It helps children to understand that their feelings are normal, including the way they feel anxiety in their bodies. Teaching a child to say "My tummy feels fluttery when I try new things, and that is just my body's way of saying to pay attention to whether or not I like it," or "My muscles get tight when I'm scared, and that is my body's way of preparing to run and get help if I need to" benefits anxious kids (and grown-ups, too).

What Coping with Anxiety Can Look Like in Real Life

Aisha is successful at her job. Her work output is double that of her coworkers, and she receives praise from her boss for her work quality. However, she feels like it isn't good enough and continuously feels self-doubt and pressure to perform better. She expects perfection from herself, and she has a hard time reconciling when she feels like she has made a mistake or could have done something "better." As a result, she puts in long hours at work and rarely allows herself to take a day off. She never feels like she can rest, as her mind always seems to keep going. At night, her thoughts are even louder, which makes it difficult to fall asleep. In the morning, she jumps right into work mode, and is checking emails even before she gets out of bed. She finds herself feeling drained, and only seems to have energy to zone out on her phone.

After feeling this way for months, she decides to reach out to a therapist. She can't keep on going at this pace. Her therapist helps her to explore the expectations she has of herself, and she acknowledges how unrealistic they are. She works on creating a sense of identity apart from work. She doesn't want her self-worth to be tied to the feedback she gets from her boss. She leans into finding success and happiness in a different, healthier way.

When she finds her anxiety starting to build, she uses the breathing exercises her therapist suggested and notices her body and brain starting to relax. She also starts challenging her negative self-talk. The thought *I'm not good enough* is one that pops up often. During those tough therapy sessions when it feels impossible to be kind to herself, her therapist reminds her that it's a marathon and not a sprint. She's working to undo years of learned self-talk and negative beliefs about herself. Progress, not perfection has become her new mantra.

READING LIST AND OTHER RESOURCES

Self-Compassion: The Proven Power of Being Kind to Yourself by Kristin Neff will help you understand the scientific basis for and life-changing potential of the practice of self-compassion.

Anxiety Rx: A New Prescription for Anxiety Relief from the Doctor Who Created It by Russell Kennedy explores anxiety's mind-body connection and teaches ways to rewire anxiety throughout the body. Prefer to listen to a podcast? You can listen to an interview where Kennedy describes his approach to anxiety on episode 183 of *The Liz Moody Podcast.*

The Perfectionism Journal: Guided Prompts and Mindfulness Practices to Reduce Anxiety and Find Calm by Tina Kocol. This book provides journal prompts and exercises to help you get into touch with your expectations of perfectionism and guide you in creating a healthier relationship with yourself.

The Gifts of Imperfection: Let Go of Who You Think You're Supposed to Be and Embrace Who You Are by Brené Brown is a powerful book about the impact of feeling a need to be perfect and exploring the freedom in letting go of that narrative.

A Happier You by Scott Glassman helps you to connect with positivity and building resiliency by following a seven-week program of actionable steps to transform your thinking.

Accessing the Healing Power of the Vagus Nerve by Stanley Rosenberg. This book helps you understand the role the vagus nerve plays in stress and anxiety, and it provides exercises for increasing the resilience of the vagus nerve.

Burnout: The Secret to Unlocking the Stress Cycle by Emily and Amelia Nagoski helps you understand how stress lives in the body and how to release it through discharge.

Trauma Sensitive Mindfulness by David Treleaven can help if you're trying to learn more about mindfulness and meditation but have a trauma or mental health history that makes it difficult for you to sit still and focus.

Feel, Deal, Heal is a coping card deck designed by therapist Tiffany Roe that aims to help you safely connect with your feelings and learn to tolerate them, an approach that is helpful for anxiety of all kinds.

Mindfulness Coach is an app created by the Department of Veterans Affairs that walks you through basic mindfulness exercises, including one of our favorites, Leaves on a Stream.

Breathe2Relax, iBreathe, and Breath Ball are free apps designed to help you take a moment to breathe and calm your anxiety.

Calm and Headspace are subscription-based apps designed to help you work through your anxiety in the moment as well as improve your quality of sleep, ability to focus, and more.

IFS Guide is an app that can help you get to know and befriend your anxiety through a "parts lens," teaching you to look at how different parts of yourself take on roles to protect you from difficult emotions or experiences—like an inner critic that makes you work harder before someone else can criticize you.

 "Elmo's Belly Breathing" is a child-friendly YouTube video that can help guide kids through breathing exercises.

 Meditation Is an Open Sky: Mindfulness for Kids by Whitney Stewart is a children's book that does a lovely job teaching kids about mindfulness and visualization practices.

 Listening to My Body by Gabi Garcia teaches both kids and grown-ups how to notice and listen to what your body is trying to communicate.

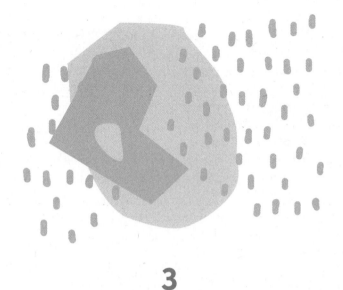

3

GENERALIZED ANXIETY DISORDER

You probably worry sometimes, as this is a normal part of the human condition. Worry can help you consider possible future outcomes and feel prepared in case something goes wrong. Nevertheless, there is a point at which worrying stops being productive, slows your progress, and leads to significant anxiety.

A helpful way to think about worry is that it's like a smoke detector. Smoke detectors are necessary to protect us from danger, but if yours is going off all the time, you may find it to be a nuisance and may even disconnect it. In this chapter, we hope to teach you ways to make the most of your worry without it driving you up a wall (or tempting you to disconnect it from the wall altogether!).

When your worry becomes distressing and disruptive to your daily life, you may be diagnosed with Generalized Anxiety Disorder (GAD). A generalized worry means you worry about many things and the focus of the worry changes. You may worry about your finances, work, or relationships.

> **THE RESEARCH SAYS . . .**
>
> ## You Are Not Alone
> GAD affects approximately 6.2 percent of people around the world.[2]

Generalized Anxiety Disorder is diagnosed based on the following criteria.[1]

- You experience excessive anxiety and worry (apprehensive expectation), occurring more often than not for at least six months, about a number of events or activities (such as work or school performance).

- You find it difficult to control the worry.

- Your anxiety and worry are associated with three or more of the following six symptoms, with at least some of the symptoms being present more often than not for the past six months: restlessness or feeling keyed up or on edge, being easily fatigued, difficulty concentrating or mind going blank, irritability, muscle tension, or sleep disturbance (difficulty falling or staying asleep, or restless, unsatisfying sleep).

- The anxiety, worry, or physical symptoms cause you clinically significant distress or impairment in your social or occupational life, or in other important areas of functioning.

You may have learned that the best way to keep yourself safe and perform well (such as at work or school) is to be cautious and worry. However, the worry is likely having a negative effect on your performance, potentially creating a negative self-fulfilling prophecy: a belief about yourself or an outcome that you then act on consciously or unconsciously, validating the belief. For example, you may believe that you'll do poorly on a test. That belief and anxiety leads you to either avoid studying or not retain the information while you're attempting to study, because your negative prediction keeps popping up ("Why even bother? I'm going to fail anyway"), the end result being you do poorly on the test. It is important to recognize when worrying is no longer helping you and to instead use positive coping strategies to prepare for the future.

What Professional Help May Look Like

COGNITIVE BEHAVIORAL THERAPY

Cognitive Behavioral Therapy (CBT) and applied relaxation can help reduce your GAD symptoms.[3] CBT can even help address any symptoms of depression you may experience alongside GAD.[4] It can also help you better cope with feelings of uncertainty.[5]

CBT helps you change the patterns of thinking that lead to anxiety. You challenge thoughts that assume actions are riskier than they are, and therefore change your catastrophic thinking (which is when you expect the worst outcome will happen).[6]

You also learn Cognitive Restructuring strategies to reframe your negative thoughts to become more balanced and realistic, which may be helpful in managing your anxiety-provoking thoughts and mental imagery.[7]

MINDFULNESS-BASED STRESS REDUCTION

Mindfulness-Based Stress Reduction (MBSR) helps you learn to focus your attention on the present, acknowledge your emotions, and use meditation strategies to further reduce stress.[8] Mindfulness often includes moment-to-moment awareness, taking a nonjudgmental approach to your thoughts, meditation techniques, and daily practice. (See chapter 2 for practical mindfulness strategies.)

MEDICATION

Medication, like selective serotonin reuptake inhibitors (SSRIs), may also help GAD.[9] SSRIs include medications such as citalopram, escitalopram, fluoxetine, fluvoxamine, paroxetine, and sertraline. It is recommended that

---

THE RESEARCH SAYS . . .

This Is How GAD Affects Your Brain and Body

If you have GAD, you may have overactivity in the parts of your brain related to threat-response. Specifically, dysfunction may be present in the circuitry that supports mental processes, such as attention, emotion, learning, and memory.[10]

Often, the body is the first place where anxiety manifests, although we don't always realize that at the time. GAD has also been linked to headaches, joint pain, and dizziness.[11] Learning to notice the early signs that your body is displaying anxiety can help you begin to practice coping strategies before the anxiety becomes too intense.

such medication be continued for at least one year to reduce the likelihood of GAD symptoms returning,[12] although you should consult with your clinician about what is best for you.

Strategies to Try

PRACTICE MINDFULNESS

Practicing mindfulness strategies can help soothe feelings of nervousness or irritability. This could involve taking a few moments to take a deep breath and notice what you see, hear, touch, smell, and taste. The goal is not to judge what you are perceiving but simply to notice. This can soothe the tension you may be carrying in your body and give a brief reprieve from your worries. You can increase the soothing benefits of this practice by focusing on something you find calming, such as a cup of herbal tea, going outside in nature, or playing with a pet.

IDENTIFY AND REFRAME YOUR UNHELPFUL THOUGHTS

If you are worried that you won't succeed, it may be helpful to recognize the fears connected to that thought. Sometimes your mind will jump several steps ahead and make negative predictions. Your worry about getting a bad grade on a paper may lead to a fear that you will fail the class, be kicked out of school, and not be able to pay back your student loans. The anxiety you feel may be understandable if it is connected to such a big cost. See if you can figure out how the worry is trying to help or protect you. Noticing and validating the positive intention of the worry often gives you enough space to change your perspective.

It can also be helpful to challenge these assumptions, such as getting kicked out of school. If you fail a class, it's likely that you will be able to retake it. It may be helpful to reassure yourself that you do not need to be perfect, that the people who care about you will still love you even if you fail a class, and that avoidance is only fueling your anxiety.

Ask yourself, "Will this still matter in six months, five years, twenty years?" This can help you recognize that although the worry may feel big right now, very few worries will still matter in time.

TURN YOUR "WHAT-IF" THOUGHTS INTO "TO-DO" THOUGHTS

Identify which thoughts are "what-if" thoughts. Catch the thoughts that cause you worry about what could happen if something goes wrong. For each thought, make a list of things you can do to address the worry. "What if I get a flat tire?" Have a spare in your trunk.

If your "what-if" thought persists after turning it into a "to-do," you will want to further process the underlying related fears and beliefs with a therapist.

USE GUIDED IMAGERY

You can use Guided Imagery as a relaxation technique to activate your senses and soothe and reduce your anxiety through imagining pleasing places, events, or objects.[13] You can have a professional lead you through it, follow a recording, or create your own.[14]

PRACTICE INTEROCEPTION

Learning and practicing body-based strategies can be helpful to shift your experience of anxiety from inaccurately interpreting your bodily sensations to accurately interpreting them and responding to them appropriately. For example, this means recognizing that when you have a mildly upset stomach, the thought *This means something is terribly wrong with me* is unfounded; instead, you're able to tell yourself *My upset stomach is a symptom of anxiety, and as I take slow, deep breaths, the feeling will fade*. Start by learning to notice and interpret what your body is communicating with you, a practice called "interoception."

Strengthening your interoception could begin with tasks such as noticing and attending to your body when it is hungry, thirsty, or needs the bathroom. Building a relationship with your body communicates that you are a willing listener to its cues, and that you will take action based on them. This becomes important when using body-based strategies, such as breathing exercises, to try and communicate back to your body to feel calm.

You could also participate in more formal body-based experiences such as biofeedback or yoga. Practicing yoga even once a week can decrease anxiety.[15] You can learn to interpret an increased heart rate not as something that will harm you, but as something you can regulate through slowing your breathing. If you can accurately interpret what your body is saying to you, then you can more rationally approach your worried thoughts.[16]

Barriers to Feeling Better

WORRIES WITH BIG IMPLICATIONS CAN BE HARD TO REFRAME

You may find it difficult to reframe worries that feel riskier. For example, there could be a big cost to your financial stability if you get fired. It could make it harder to appear qualified for the "perfect" future job and threaten your financial stability.

It is still possible to reframe and find alternative thoughts for these worries (for example, you could get unemployment or live with family). However, it can be more difficult to fully believe these reframes or feel completely soothed. In these situations, the worry is often connected to core beliefs we have about ourselves, others, and the world around us. CBT is helpful in recognizing the roots of such worry.

Practicing self-compassion for those parts of us that are concerned about such big consequences is helpful as well. If you can find the core belief beneath your worry, then you can offer it compassion in a meaningful way. For example, if the root of your anxiety is the fear that *if you aren't successful, you won't be loved*, you can offer yourself the compassion to say, "I will always love myself no matter if I succeed or not."

THE TWENTY-FOUR-HOUR NEWS CYCLE

It's impossible not to experience stress or anxiety at times, given how the news cycle highlights catastrophes locally and around the world, and the internet makes news constantly accessible. If our anxiety results in us hyperfocusing on the negative, then we can start to feel hopeless and depressed.

News outlets, advertisers, and social networking platforms know

---

THE RESEARCH SAYS . . .

You May Also Experience These Things

If you have GAD, you are more likely to be diagnosed with Obsessive-Compulsive Disorder, Post-Traumatic Stress Disorder (page 57), and specific phobias, such as a fear of heights or animals.[17]

The generalized nature of GAD means it can overlap with other illnesses. If you have Illness Anxiety Disorder, you often worry about acquiring an illness. If you have Social Anxiety Disorder, you worry about being negatively evaluated by others, but that fear can manifest in all types of situations (such as speaking in class or while checking out at the store). Of note, you can have GAD, Illness Anxiety Disorder, and Social Anxiety Disorder simultaneously; they are not mutually exclusive.

that messages causing us to feel angry or scared are more effective. This means that the "reality" created online is not often a true picture of the world.

It is difficult, although extremely healthy, to take breaks from social media and the news. If you can't do this for long periods of time, experiment with the short-term, such as an hour before you go to bed every night, or one day each weekend. Notice if you feel more relaxed during your news and social media breaks.

There are times that accepting your anxiety is the healthiest approach. For example, when it is warning you about the catastrophic implications of climate change or war, it's healthy to recognize and soothe your anxiety, but not to try and talk yourself out of it.

How to Communicate About GAD

IF YOU'RE THE ONE DEALING WITH GAD

Tell others when you are feeling overwhelmed and express to them how they can help you in the moment. If you don't feel comfortable telling someone else about your worry, then be sure to use relaxation techniques to reduce your physical sensations of stress and then use general terms to tell the other person what you need from them, saying something like, "I need a moment to gather my thoughts." If you need to, step into the bathroom or another private room to do some breathing or grounding exercises before coming back and attempting to reconnect with others.

IF A LOVED ONE IS DEALING WITH GAD

Ask them how you can best provide support without minimizing their worry or taking a "fix it" approach. Telling someone with GAD that "it will be fine" or to "just stop worrying" may have limited effect on their worry and may lead them to avoid confiding in you in the future. Let your loved one know you are there to listen if they want to process their worry out loud. Ask them if they are looking for you to help them with problem solving or if they simply want you to empathize with them about how stressful the situation is.

IF THE PERSON DEALING WITH GAD IS A CHILD

It's important to remember that children do not always express their anxiety the same way adults do. Children often express GAD through physiological symptoms, such as by saying they have an upset stomach.[18] It is important to avoid judgmental statements or language comparing your child to another as they may be risk-averse, perfectionistic, and seek constant reassurance.[19]

Notice if they show avoidance or tend to say they feel physically ill when either discussing or being asked to engage in potentially stressful activities.

What Coping with Generalized Anxiety Disorder Can Look Like in Real Life

Lee is a full-time parent, juggling taking care of their kids with taking care of their aging parents and their own chronic health issues. Over the past year, they've noticed that they have started to feel more stressed throughout the day. They are often clenching their jaw and tensing their shoulders. They've been having trouble concentrating on tasks and find it difficult to stay asleep at night. They have started worrying more than ever and the focus of the worry shifts depending on what they are thinking about.

Lee decides to see their primary care clinician. The clinician asks them to complete some questionnaires and tells them that they could have Generalized Anxiety Disorder (GAD), but it also could be Obsessive-Compulsive Disorder, Social Anxiety Disorder, or Attention-Deficit/Hyperactivity Disorder. The clinician offers to do some blood work to check things like their thyroid and offers to start them on an SSRI for anxiety. The clinician encourages Lee to speak with a therapist for a full clinical interview (questions regarding their past and current experiences) or even an assessment (multiple tests interpreted by a psychologist) to home in on a diagnosis.

Lee sees a therapist who helps them rule out other diagnoses and identify that they are likely dealing with GAD. They ask Lee to write down stressful situations and their accompanying thoughts, feelings, and behaviors each day. This helps them notice patterns in what causes their anxiety. They practice reframing their negative thoughts to come up with ones that are more balanced and realistic. Lee has learned to turn their "what-if" thoughts into "to-do" thoughts, and to recognize that there may be a bigger worry or negative belief related to the thought when they continue to worry after completing all the related "to-dos."

The relaxation and mindfulness strategies they have worked on, including guided imagery and 4-7-8 breathing exercises, have helped them self-soothe, and Lee even teaches the strategies to their kids. Like their therapist taught them, they breathe in slowly through their nose to a count of 4, and gently hold it for a count of 7. Then they slowly let the breath out through their mouth to a count of 8. At the bottom of their breath, they exhale just a little more to make sure they've fully released their breath. They want to get all of the breath out, and then repeat.

After a few months, Lee still experiences daily worry, but that worry does not get in the way of them being fully engaged in their tasks and relationships. They've learned to appreciate their worry for what it's trying to do for them and then shift how they approach it.

READING LIST AND OTHER RESOURCES

The Cognitive Behavioral Workbook for Anxiety: A Step-By-Step Program by William J. Knaus is a workbook that walks you through some of the exercises described in this chapter, and more.

For more resources, see the list on page 29.

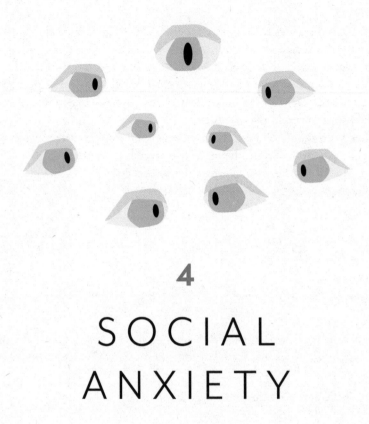

4

SOCIAL ANXIETY

Y ou may experience stress in social situations. Such feelings of excitement or anxiety can feel similar in our bodies. It's normal to worry about what others think of you, however, Social Anxiety Disorder, also known as Social Phobia, occurs when you feel intense fear or anxiety related to how you think you will be viewed by others. You worry that you may act in a way that will be perceived negatively, which may ultimately lead to your exclusion.

Social Anxiety Disorder is diagnosed based on the following criteria.[1]

- You feel marked fear or anxiety about one or more social situations in which you are exposed to possible scrutiny (critical observation) by others.

- You fear you will act in a way or show anxiety symptoms that will be humiliating or embarrassing, negatively evaluated, and/or will lead to rejection from or offend others.

- Being in social situations almost always provokes fear or anxiety in you, and you avoid or endure them with intense fear or anxiety.

- Your fear or anxiety is out of proportion to the actual threat posed by the situation.

- Your fear, anxiety, or avoidance is persistent, typically lasting six months or more.

- You can experience a performance-only type of Social Anxiety Disorder if the fear is restricted to speaking or performing in public.

- The anxiety, worry, or physical symptoms cause you clinically significant distress or impairment in social or occupational life, or in other important areas of functioning.

When anxious, you may avoid stressful situations, because fleeing a potential threat is a response that often keeps you safe. For example, if you are worried about how people will look at you when you're at the store, then you just don't go to the store. From that you learn that the only way to protect yourself from possible external judgment is to stay home. You don't get the chance to learn that most people won't judge you, they likely will be focused on themselves, and even if they did make judgments, it has no real impact on your life. (If this sounds like you and you've become lonely as a result, you may also benefit from reading chapter 11.)

Some may have a tough time in social settings and prefer relationships in small settings or online. If you know that unpredictable social situations aren't good for you, this chapter doesn't aim to change you. However, if you are someone who wants to be more socially engaged but you find that social anxiety makes it feel impossible, read on.

THE RESEARCH SAYS . . .

You Are Not Alone

Approximately 12 percent of Americans will experience Social Anxiety Disorder in their lifetime, with the average age of onset being thirteen.[2]

What Professional Help May Look Like

COGNITIVE BEHAVIORAL THERAPY

Cognitive Behavioral Therapy (CBT) is an effective treatments for children, adolescents, and adults with Social Anxiety Disorder.[3] Incorporating social skills practice into such therapy is especially helpful.

A cognitive focus in therapy can guide you to recognize when you are holding negative thoughts about yourself, overestimating the cost of a social mishap, thinking you have little control over your emotions, and believing that your social skills are inadequate.[4]

In CBT, you will likely be asked to safely expose yourself to the feared stimuli, either in real life or through imagined scenarios.[5] You can engage in CBT face-to-face or by computer, tablet, or smartphone application, and in some places even through virtual reality.[6]

KID-FRIENDLY TIP If your child is experiencing social anxiety, CBT can teach them how to interact with others using social skills practice.[7] Moreover, you may consider parent/caregiver therapy so that you can learn to manage your own concerns about your child's anxiety.

EXPOSURE THERAPY

Exposure helps you to change the vicious cycle of avoidance and enable new "safety learning" so that the expected bad outcome you are dreading does not occur or becomes manageable.[8] For example, each time you talk to a new person and nothing bad happens, you build more evidence that it's safe to increase your social activity.

Through Exposure Therapy, you can challenge and disprove your cognitive distortions (unhelpful thinking) related to social expectations.[9] If you fear public speaking, you may have the worried thought that you will "be mocked and seen as unprofessional," and then may avoid public speaking. The more you engage in public speaking, even to small groups, you learn that such thoughts are not facts, just unhelpful thinking habits.

Additionally, you may benefit from graded exposure to anxiety stressors.[10] This means slowly and safely going into situations that are stressful and increasing your level of comfort over time. It's important to note that Exposure Therapy is inherently uncomfortable, as it is asking you to face the very thing you fear. What will make this bearable is a safe, supportive relationship with the professional walking you through it. (Check out chapter 24 if you need guidance on connecting with the right therapist for you.)

MEDICATION

If you decline to engage in talk therapy, selective serotonin reuptake inhibitors (SSRIs) and selective norepinephrine reuptake inhibitors (SNRIs), show the most consistent evidence to help relieve symptoms if you have Social Anxiety Disorder.[11] Medication alone (SSRIs and SNRIs) or the combination of CBT and medication can be helpful.[12]

Strategies to Try

PRACTICE GRADED EXPOSURE

You can slowly and safely build your confidence in social situations through graded exposure. If you experience high levels of distress during certain activities, it will be especially helpful to engage in this following strategy while working with a therapist. You start by creating a list of the social situations (such as talking to a stranger at the store or asking someone for directions) that make you feel stressed and rate each of them on their Subjective Units of Distress (SUDs), from 0 to 10; 0 being not stressful at all and 10 being the most intense level of stress. After writing down and rating all your stressful situations, copy them into a list from least to most stressful. Next, starting with the least stressful situations, put yourself in each of them one by one.

You can start with imaginal exposure (thinking about what the social situation would be like), then work your way to doing the activity in real life. The goal is to approach the stressful situation slowly, while using healthy self-soothing and relaxation techniques, and reduce your SUDs, hopefully to 0 for each item, or at least to a functional level like 1 or 2.

KID-FRIENDLY TIP Kids can make SUDs scales and stressful situation hierarchies, too! Have them use fun materials like paper and crayons to make their list. Or have them use a chalk or white board; this way they can change the SUDs as their experiences of anxiety change.

The more we build evidence that we can successfully navigate and manage our anxiety in social situations, the less stressful that situation becomes.

Of course, if your worry is helping protect you from a real threat, don't try to reframe it! Listen to it and respect the message it is giving you. By learning when to listen to our anxiety and when to reframe it, we are building a relationship with it, a first step to befriending it.

TRY PROGRESSIVE MUSCLE RELAXATION

You may find Progressive Muscle Relaxation helpful in reducing physical sensations of stress.[13] When learning the technique, a clinician will guide you through the muscle groups where you carry tension. You will be asked to skip tensing any muscle groups where added tension may lead you to feel pain. You will tense a muscle group (like your shoulders or hands) for about eight to ten seconds, then release the tension and notice the difference between the sensations of relaxation and tension.

Barriers to Feeling Better

NEGATIVE PAST EXPERIENCES

Anxiety can be protective as your worries can be focused on big areas of concern. It's harder to break a cycle of anxiety if the social situation you fear comes from past bad experiences, such as cruelty from others or if you've been negatively evaluated. You may have experienced bullying or received a bad grade for a speech you had to give in school. Such experiences can fuel unhelpful thoughts and you may benefit from therapy to process the past negative experiences.

MIND READING

Assuming you know what others are thinking about you, or "mind reading," is an unhelpful thinking habit. Mind reading can be adaptive, as it's helpful to have a sense of how people are responding to you during a conversation. However, it becomes unhelpful when you assume they are thinking negatively when they haven't given any such indication.

OVERGENERALIZATION

Overgeneralization occurs when you worry that bad things will consistently happen to you in the future ("I will mess up *every* time I give a speech") because you had a similar negative experience in the past (forgetting your speech in the middle of a presentation). You may find it helpful to think about past speeches and what you did well each time. This can help you build evidence toward a more balanced thought.

MAKING NEGATIVE PREDICTIONS

Negative predictions involve thinking that a specific future event will have a negative outcome, when in reality you don't have any concrete evidence to back it up. For example, to convince yourself not to talk to new people at a party, you may think *They will laugh at me if I talk to them.*

To reframe these thoughts, it can be beneficial to ask yourself the following questions.

- What's the worst that could happen?
- Could I live through it?
- Are there still people who love and support me?
- If someone I cared about was having this thought, what would I tell them?

THE RESEARCH SAYS . . .

You May Also Experience These Things

If you have Social Anxiety Disorder, you may also be more likely to experience Obsessive-Compulsive Disorder, Post-Traumatic Stress Disorder (page 57), and specific phobias, such as a fear of heights or animals.[14] Additionally, it has overlapping symptoms with Panic Disorder (page 48), Agoraphobia, atypical depression, and body dysmorphia (page 173).[15]

How to Communicate About Social Anxiety

IF YOU'RE THE ONE EXPERIENCING SOCIAL ANXIETY

Talk through your worries with trusted loved ones. Tell them about your discomfort and ask for their support when entering social situations. You may say, "I'll come to this event with you, but I'd like for us to sit together at least until I am feeling comfortable." Others may not know about your worries until you tell them, so be brave and ask for the support you need in an effort to reduce your avoidance of social situations.

IF A LOVED ONE IS EXPERIENCING SOCIAL ANXIETY

If it is their goal, gently encourage them to go into situations that can help them increase their positive social experiences. However, it is important not to push them faster than they are comfortable with, and to support them throughout the process. Ask "How can I best support you?" and reassure them with "I will stay with you." If your loved one is happy with their current level of social interaction, respect that.

IF THE PERSON EXPERIENCING SOCIAL ANXIETY IS A CHILD

Make sure their social anxiety is not coming from a real concern that needs to be addressed, such as bullying, harassment, or even abuse. Children and even teenagers often don't have the words for bad things that are happening to them. Refusal to participate in a social situation could be the only way they know how to protect themselves.

If your child doesn't want to talk to you about it, you can help them identify safe people they can share their fears or concerns with, such as another family member, a teacher, or a therapist.

What Coping with Social Anxiety Can Look Like in Real Life

Jory has been asked to give a presentation at a conference on behalf of their work. The presentation means they will need to speak in front of a room of fifty people. They are terrified of giving speeches in front of large crowds, as they know from past experiences that they get sweaty, red, and trip over their words. Jory is afraid that people will notice how nervous they look and will think they're unqualified for their position, and may even think poorly of their employer for hiring them.

Knowing that they must give this presentation, Jory goes to see their primary care clinician. The clinician talks with Jory about possible medication to help them get through the speech that day, but cautions that the medication may not be the only solution, as it comes with side effects, and they'd need to be mindful about how it could negatively impact their speech-giving abilities. While Jory is considering medication, they are also referred to a therapist to discuss Cognitive Behavior Therapy strategies. The cognitive model of how their thoughts, feelings, and behaviors impact each other resonates with them and they start to notice the worried thoughts they are having about giving the presentation. They identify the unhelpful thoughts: *I will mess this up for everyone*, and *People will laugh at me.*

The therapist teaches Jory relaxation techniques, including deep breathing and Progressive Muscle Relaxation (PMR). They find that they enjoy PMR, which is an exercise where they slowly tense and then release different muscle groups in their body. Jory also begins to engage in exposure activities to help them build confidence in their speaking abilities and reduce their level of stress related to speech-giving activities. They practice recording the speech and watching themself, and they present the speech to their family. With each exposure activity and repeat practice, Jory's level of stress lowers. By utilizing deep breathing, exposure strategies, challenging their negative thoughts, and trialing a medication, they are able to give the presentation and even get positive feedback.

READING LIST AND OTHER RESOURCES

The Shyness and Social Anxiety Workbook: Proven, Step-by-Step Techniques for Overcoming Your Fear by Martin M. Antony and Richard P. Swinson can provide you with strategies to reduce your avoidance and increase your confidence in building relationships.

The National Social Anxiety Center (nationalsocialanxietycenter.com) provides several free education and skills-building resources to help manage social anxiety.

For more resources, see the list on page 29.

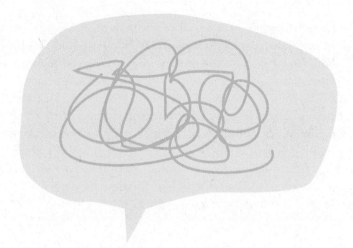

5

PANIC DISORDER

I f you have a panic attack you may experience symptoms such as a pound-ing heart, an upset stomach, or tightness in your chest. These symptoms can often be explained by common occurrences, such as going for a run, having a cold, or being outside during a heatwave. However, when many of these symptoms overlap, it may also mean that you are experiencing a panic attack or even Panic Disorder. Panic attacks come out of nowhere, but they can be connected to a thought or physical sensation. For example, your heart skips a beat, provoking you to worry that you may be dying. That thought may then cause your stress to increase, causing more panic-like symptoms to occur and overlap.

Panic attacks can negatively impact your functioning and increase your risk for various other mental disorders.[1] If you're experiencing panic attacks or Panic Disorder, you may feel like you are having a heart attack. It is not uncommon to feel exhausted or even sick for hours to days after a panic attack, particularly an intense one. It's important during this recovery time to recognize your limits, engage in good self-care, and be kind to yourself.

You may likely seek treatment for panic symptoms in primary care, cardiology, or the emergency room, where the diagnosis is more often missed than in psychiatric care.[2] If sought treatment focuses primarily on medical concerns, it can increase the risk of Panic Disorder being missed and assumed to be a heart problem, which may result in invasive and unneeded testing.

The reality is that no one would advise you against seeking medical attention if you think you are having a heart attack. It's important to recognize that Panic Disorder is a complicated diagnosis to pull apart from other medical conditions, it can be diagnosed in people who have no other health diagnoses, and it should always be taken seriously. If diagnosed with Panic Disorder, you may find that you are likely to feel more easily stressed when facing a generic threat (such as being cut off while driving), but also have increased sensitivity for specific threat contents (such as feeling short of breath) related to your panic attacks.[3]

Panic Disorder is diagnosed based on the following criteria.[4]

- You experience repeat unexpected panic attacks. A panic attack is an abrupt surge of intense fear or discomfort that reaches a peak within minutes and during which time you experience at least four of the following symptoms: palpitations, pounding heart, or accelerated heart rate; sweating; trembling or shaking; sensations of shortness of breath or smothering; feelings of choking; chest pain or discomfort; nausea or abdominal distress; feeling dizzy, unsteady, lightheaded, or faint; chills or heat sensations; paresthesia (numbness or tingling sensations); derealization (feelings of unreality) or depersonalization (feeling detached from yourself); fear of losing control or "going crazy"; or fear of dying.

- At least one of your panic attacks has been followed by a month or longer of you being persistently concerned or worried about additional panic attacks or their consequences (for example, having a heart attack), or of you experiencing a significant maladaptive change in behavior related to the attacks (such as avoidance of a behavior in an effort not to have a panic attack).

- Your anxiety, worry, or physical symptoms cause you clinically significant distress or impairment in your social or occupational life, or in other important areas of functioning.

What Professional Help May Look Like

COGNITIVE BEHAVIORAL THERAPY

You may benefit from CBT, as it is an effective treatment for Panic Disorder,[6] through guided self-help or face-to-face therapy.[7]

You will likely learn through CBT that after having a panic attack, you may form Panic Disorder due to a misinterpretation of the symptoms (believing your pounding heart means you are having a heart attack), starting a cycle in which such negative thoughts lead to physical symptoms (lightheadedness), which then may result in a panic attack and more thoughts that something bad is happening (for example, "I'm dying").[8] You may doubt your ability to cope with the physical symptoms, causing continued feelings of anxiety and panic.[9]

INTEROCEPTIVE EXPOSURE

If treated with CBT, you may be taught a technique called Interoceptive Exposure. It involves you purposefully causing the physical sensations related to having a panic attack.[10] For example, you may increase your heart rate by running or hyperventilating to disprove the idea that the physical sensations associated with a panic attack will lead to harmful events such as a heart attack. As this is an intense experience, it's best done with a qualified mental health professional.

MEDICATION

You may benefit from the combination of CBT and medication rather than medication alone, but engaging in just CBT still provides similar benefits.[11] Therefore, starting a medication can be considered if your Panic Disorder is long-standing, or you have not benefited from or have declined talk therapy.

You may consider talking with your clinician about selective serotonin reuptake inhibitors (SSRIs) or benzodiazepines for your Panic Disorder, as they are often the medications considered first.[12] SSRIs, like sertraline and escitalopram, tend to be associated with higher benefit and lower side effects.[13]

It's important that you are aware that benzodiazepines may be effective in a short-term crisis, however long-term use of these medicines is associated with dependence and higher rate of mortality (including higher suicide risk), so clinicians are cautioned from prescribing them.[14]

Talk to your clinician about the pros and cons of any type of treatment, especially with certain medications, like benzodiazepines. Overall, you may choose medication to treat your Panic Disorder but it needs to be discussed thoroughly with a health care clinician and taken with an understanding of the potential risks.

Strategies to Try

REMIND YOURSELF THAT THE PANIC ATTACK WILL END

Symptoms of panic reach a peak within minutes and then subside. This fact can be reassuring. Panic attacks, by definition, do not last a long time. A strategy for coping with panic can include reminding yourself of this fact. Such phrases as "I can get through this" and "This feels bad, but it won't last forever" may be helpful. Some people find it useful to set a timer for a few minutes and remind themselves that when the timer goes off, their panic will have subsided.

WATCH SAFE DEPICTIONS OF PANIC AND ANXIETY

Sometimes, depictions of panic attacks in movies or TV shows can help normalize them for kids who need to know that their panic attack will end. The movie *Puss In Boots: The Last Wish* depicts panic attacks, and the movies *Frozen, Finding Nemo*, and *Toy Story* show examples of intense anxiety.

"SAFETY BEHAVIORS" MAY REDUCE THE PANIC, BUT DON'T DEPEND ON THEM

You may be encouraged to utilize relaxation techniques when experiencing symptoms of panic. Taking deep breaths or tensing and relaxing muscle groups are "safety behaviors" that may help you cope. Nevertheless, the ultimate goal is often to be able to sit through a panic attack without trying to reduce or avoid the symptoms, or by using "safety behaviors." Safety habits, like slowing your breath, help you let time pass, which is the biggest component in helping the panic attack pass. Getting through a panic attack is easier said than done. Therefore, there is nothing wrong with using healthy coping strategies to manage the panic as you work on exposure techniques and CBT strategies to improve your confidence to sit through the feelings of panic.

It is okay to use safety behaviors, and you may choose to do so long-term, though once you are able to reduce the length of the panic attack and your related feelings of distress, it may be beneficial to start to delay or decrease their use. It helps to build evidence that the panic symptoms are not life threatening and you can get through them. Doing so ensures you are able to "ride the wave" of the panic attack no matter where you are and what safety items you have available, helping your panic in the long term. Ultimately, you decide what helps you feel safe.

Barriers to Feeling Better

THE DIFFICULTY OF DIAGNOSING A PANIC ATTACK

Because Panic Disorder can overlap with several medical and mental health diagnoses, it can be difficult to recognize the diagnosis, let alone engage in evidence-based treatment for it. The physical symptoms of panic attacks can look like other diagnoses that should not be ignored, as they could be life threatening. However, sometimes this overlap can make it difficult for you to fully accept reassurance from your medical clinician that there is nothing wrong physically.

Frequent visits to medical clinics or the emergency room due to panic attacks and/or Panic Disorder can result in medical clinicians missing more complex medical diagnoses. There is a common saying in medical training that most diagnoses are horses (common), not zebras (rare). Based on statistics, this is true, but it can result in clinicians missing the rarer diagnoses, especially with panic attacks clouding the picture.

While Panic Disorder is a diagnosis that stands on its own, panic attacks can be present in many other mental health diagnoses. For example, you can have Social Anxiety Disorder or Post-Traumatic Stress Disorder, both with panic attacks. In such cases, the cause of the panic attacks is related to these other diagnoses. To be diagnosed with Panic Disorder, the cause of your anxiety needs to be the panic attacks themselves—a subtle but important distinction.

THE RESEARCH SAYS . . .

You May Also Experience These Things

If you have Panic Disorder, you are more likely to also have Coronary Artery Disease, with the prevalence ranging from 10 to 50 percent in this subgroup.[17]

If you have panic attacks and/or Panic Disorder, you may also experience Agoraphobia, Social Anxiety Disorder (page 40), Generalized Anxiety Disorder (page 31), Major Depressive Disorder (page 9), Persistent Depressive Disorder, Bipolar Disorder, and Alcohol Use Disorder (page 189).[18] 48 to 68 percent of adults who have one anxiety disorder also meet criteria to be simultaneously diagnosed with another.[19]

How to Communicate About Panic Disorder

IF YOU'RE THE ONE DEALING WITH PANIC DISORDER

Tell others what helps you cope when you experience panic symptoms and ask them to support you by reminding you of your positive coping thoughts. If you want them to stay present during your panic attacks, let them know and tell them coping statements to share with you, such as "You are almost through this."

If you'd prefer to be alone when you are experiencing a panic attack, let them know that, too. Explain that there may be times when you need to remove yourself from the situation to self-soothe. When you are ready, tell them what they can do to help you decrease avoidance of situations that induce panic or panic symptoms.

If you have a challenging time speaking during a panic attack, consider making your loved one aware of this and encourage them to ask you questions that can be easily answered with a nod or shake of the head.

You may also find it helpful to establish code words or hand gestures with your loved one, particularly if a panic attack were to occur while you were outside of your home, to make sure you get the support you need in the moment.

IF A LOVED ONE IS DEALING WITH PANIC DISORDER

Ask them how you can best be a support. Be mindful not to minimize their symptoms but also, when they tell you they are ready, encourage them not to avoid panic-inducing situations. Listen to their needs and ask them how you can help them feel safe while aiding them to move forward. This can be a slow process and it is most important that the person feels heard and understood. Do your best to meet them where they are.

IF THE PERSON DEALING WITH PANIC DISORDER IS A CHILD

Helping a child understand their body's responses and learn how to "ride the wave" of what is happening is important, just as it is for adults.

While Panic Disorder is rare among children, it increases in adolescence, and is particularly marked by feelings of "an unacceptable self," such as embarrassment, feeling abnormal or judged, and decreased social functioning due to the panic.[20] Because adolescents are undergoing a critical time of social development, symptoms such as panic attacks take on particular social meaning for them and should be met with empathy and understanding accordingly.

Provide education to the staff or peers in your adolescent's classroom who will be near them during a potential panic attack.[21] Give them specific phrases to say and questions to ask as your adolescent navigates their panic symptoms without leaning on "safety behaviors." A mental health professional can help you in creating phrases that are the best fit for your adolescent.

What Coping with Panic Disorder Can Look Like in Real Life

The symptoms started three months ago, shortly after Malik retired. He was driving home when he noticed his heart starting to pound. His hands felt sweaty and tingly, his vision started to blur, he found he couldn't take a deep breath, and he thought he might pass out. This scared Malik so much that he needed to pull over to the side of the road and call 911. He thought maybe his age was finally catching up to him. An ambulance came and examined him on the spot. They told him that his vitals looked normal and they could find no cause for concern. They suggested that he may have had a panic attack.

Since then, Malik has had two to three panic attacks a week. They seem to come out of nowhere and each time, he feels like he will die or lose control of his mind. He subsequently saw his primary care clinician and they told him that they could start him on a daily medication that may help, but it would likely be wise to engage in therapy to treat the root of the panic.

He attends an appointment with a therapist who tells him that the panic he is experiencing is a way for his body to keep him safe. They explain that Malik's level of stress may be connected to his thoughts and fears that the panic symptoms are dangerous. He works with the therapist on noticing the unhelpful thoughts he is having about panic, such as "I am dying" and "I won't get through this."

They help Malik reframe these negative thoughts into more adaptive thoughts: *I am okay*, and *I have gotten through each panic attack, I can keep getting through them.* He gradually starts purposefully inducing panic symptoms in his therapy sessions, by breathing quickly through a straw and running in place, in an effort to demonstrate that these symptoms (like heart pounding and shortness of breath) are not the harbingers of doom that they once seemed. After a few months, Malik notices that he is rarely having panic attacks and he does not dread the symptoms the same way he used to. He actually begins to enjoy the retirement he'd dreamed of for so long!

READING LIST AND OTHER RESOURCES

Panic Attacks Workbook: Second Edition: A Guided Program for Beating the Panic Trick, Fully Revised and Updated by David Carbonell provides insight into how panic leads you into a cycle of anticipation and helplessness, offering ways to respond to and accept panic symptoms.

The *Ten Percent Happier* podcast was created by former news anchor Dan Harris after he experienced a panic attack on air while hosting *Good Morning America*. The podcast focuses on sharing ways that the practice of mindfulness can ease our anxiety and make us happier.

For more resources, see the list on page 29.

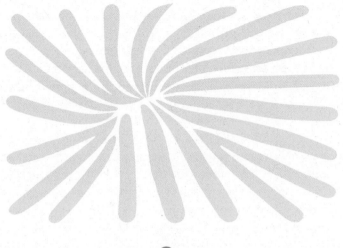

6

TRAUMA AND POST-TRAUMATIC STRESS DISORDER

This chapter discusses many aspects of trauma. If this causes you distress, be sure to read this chapter in a safe space with healthy self-soothing strategies readily available. If you find that you need to put the book down, do so. The book will be there for you when you are in a mental and emotional space to read it.

There are many definitions of trauma. We therefore find it most helpful to define "trauma" as an umbrella term, as something that overwhelms your brain and body's usual ability to cope. Trauma is not a specific type of event;

your life experiences, brain development, and internal and external resources, among other factors, will have an effect on whether an event is experienced as "trauma."[1] Two people experiencing the same event at the exact same time may process the incident differently.

You are wired for survival. Because of this, it's important to note that trauma responses are not the breakdown of your survival response, but rather your "emergency backup system."

You may be familiar with the fact that an airplane is equipped with many emergency backup systems. For example, during the preflight safety demonstration, you learn what to do in the event of an emergency. If upon hearing this you immediately pulled up and clutched the seat cushion or put on the oxygen mask, you may run the risk of being very uncomfortable.

However, if your plane had to make an emergency landing, it would be dangerous were you *not* to take those actions. In the same way, common trauma responses such as flashbacks, self-blame, and dissociation may seem useless outside of trauma, but in the aftermath, they make all the sense in the world and are your nervous system's best attempts to protect you.

Trauma is experienced by and encoded in your nervous system, which originates in your brain and spreads throughout your body through nerve cells and fibers. This means trauma is not purely a brain-based (cognitive) or body-based (somatic) experience; it is both.[2] On a daily basis, the nervous system acts like a well-oiled machine, communicating between the brain and the body in such an efficient way that you never notice it, and yet, it's making sure you breathe, allowing you to think, and even regulating your emotional experiences. In short, it's coping with life and stressful experiences all the time and re-regulating accordingly. Trauma disrupts this functioning, pushing the machine past its ability to run smoothly and self-regulate. This is when the "emergency backup system," or trauma responses, are activated. When you realize that your trauma responses are adaptive, it goes a long way to helping you let go of shame or self-blame. However, this does not mean you will enjoy them! We don't get to choose our trauma responses any more than we get to choose the trauma itself.

Helplessness is one of the most common feelings survivors of trauma experience. Because you did not choose to experience trauma, you may feel helpless about the fact that it occurred. You may also feel helpless to cope with the trauma responses your emergency backup system relies on. In this chapter, we will share ways to work with, instead of against, your nervous system's trauma responses, so that you can replace helplessness with the feeling of empowerment.

Trauma can manifest as Post-Traumatic Stress Disorder (PTSD), although not everyone will develop PTSD after experiencing a trauma.[3] The symptoms of PTSD can be broken down into four categories.

- Intrusion (you may have nightmares or flashbacks).

- Avoidance (this could be anything from conscious avoidance, or your use of intentional numbing through substances or other means, to dissociation).

- Negative alterations in cognition and mood (following a trauma you may feel self-blame, shame, and self-isolation).

- Alterations in arousal or reactivity (this includes all manifestations of hypervigilance, which can range from you having trouble sleeping, to difficulty concentrating, to a constant awareness of the surrounding environment).[4]

Even if you don't meet all the criteria for PTSD, if you're struggling with trauma you can still benefit from the following strategies. Additionally, there are other types of trauma, which are covered in chapter 7.

What Professional Help May Look Like

TRAUMA-INFORMED THERAPY

Trauma-Focused CBT and EMDR (see the following) have been found to be the most effective evidence-based therapeutic approaches to help you recover from trauma.[5]

EYE MOVEMENT DESENSITIZATION AND REPROCESSING (EMDR)

EMDR is an effective evidence-based eight-phase treatment model for trauma that allows you to reprocess your traumatic memory and construct new meaning from it.[6] Through the eight phases, you will learn resources to tolerate the distress of the traumatic memory, and with the assistance of these resources, you and your therapist target each trauma memory using a brain-based strategy called Bilateral Stimulation to reprocess it. This uses the science of memory reconsolidation to lower the distress associated with the memory and to increase your resilience and resources around it.

TRAUMA-FOCUSED COGNITIVE BEHAVIORAL THERAPY (TF-CBT)

TF-CBT is an evidence-based therapy for children.[7] It teaches the child about what trauma is, how it may be impacting them, and coping strategies that can be used. It then guides the child through the creation of a Trauma Narrative that can be completed through writing, art, or other creative ways to allow the child to process their trauma memories. TF-CBT engages the child in ways that feel familiar, like school, and therefore nonthreatening. TF-CBT has a caregiver component, so that the child's caregivers are involved in treatment every step of the way.

> **THE RESEARCH SAYS . . .**
>
> ### This Is How Trauma Can Impact Your Brain and Body
>
> Because trauma is a nervous system experience, it is held and felt throughout the body.
> You may know logically that your trauma is over, but your body is still in a perpetual state of freeze, flight, fight, or fawn that makes it feel impossible to move forward.

INTERNAL FAMILY SYSTEMS THERAPY (IFS)

IFS is a therapy approach that looks at all aspects of ourselves, including our trauma responses, as parts of self that can be befriended. The IFS model puts forth that our parts are trying to protect us, and that we can understand and have compassion for them. Working with an IFS therapist, you would be guided to get to know the parts that make up your "internal family" and release them from their burdens.[8]

TRAUMA-SENSITIVE YOGA (TSY)

Trauma-Sensitive Yoga is an evidence-based treatment for PTSD that gives you total choice over how you move your body as you are healing from trauma.[9] Unlike prescriptive yoga, TSY helps you get in touch with your body and what you need in a gentle way and in your own time.

MEDICATION

Selective serotonin reuptake inhibitors (SSRIs) can improve PTSD symptoms by reducing feelings of anxiety and fear, and some prescribers use antipsychotic medications off-label to help with symptoms of flashbacks or nightmares.[10]

Strategies to Try

GET YOURSELF GROUNDED

Grounding is one of the simplest and yet most effective trauma-informed coping strategies you can use. Simply put, grounding uses your five senses to be anchored (or grounded) in the present moment, instead of floating back to the trauma (whether through intrusive thoughts, feelings, or flashbacks). You can ground yourself using the 5-4-3-2-1 method.

- Find 5 things you see around you. Describe them in detail, either out loud or in your head. For example: I see a blanket. It is blue, square, and looks crocheted.

- Describe 4 things you can feel, such as, I can feel how soft the blanket is. I can feel my socks on my feet.

- Describe 3 things you can hear. If the room is silent, try making a sound, such as by clapping your hands or whistling.

- Describe 2 things you can smell. You may want to keep something nearby that you can use. Peppermint and coffee grounds are both grounding scents as they are strong. You may prefer a scent you enjoy and find calming.

- Describe 1 thing you can taste. Like the task above, keeping strong mints handy is useful for tasting.

Note: If any of the five senses are trauma reminders, remove them and return to something soothing.

PUT IT ON ICE

For decades, scientists have studied the mammalian dive reflex,[11] changes in the body, such as a slowed heart rate, that occur when submerged in cold water. You can induce this reflex by putting ice on your face, which calms the nervous system quickly. You may especially benefit from this if you are having a flashback, becoming dissociated, or having another intense trauma response. If that happens to you frequently, you may want to consider carrying instant cold packs, which freeze upon use.

THINK ABOUT TRAUMA RESPONSES IN TERMS OF THE WINDOW OF TOLERANCE

The term "the window of tolerance" describes the amount of arousal in which you are able to function effectively."[12] We find it helpful to think of it in terms of a river. Picture floating down a river on an inner tube. The river itself is thought of as the "optimal zone," sometimes called the "zone of living, learning, and loving." One of the shores represents the "hyperaroused zone," which is where trauma symptoms such as nightmares, flashbacks, and intense feelings live. The other shore represents the "hypoaroused zone," where trauma symptoms such as dissociation, numbness, and isolation reside.

Because trauma pushes us back and forth between these two zones, it can feel overwhelming. However, when we know that they are simply trauma responses, instead of putting all our effort into avoiding either shore, placing our focus on gradually widening the river (such as through learning coping strategies and processing trauma memories) can help us begin to live again. Knowing where we are on our own personal river, what the weather and river conditions are like on any given day, can give us the information we need to make wise and safe choices for ourselves. Eventually, you will have hours or days at a time, and eventually months and years when you are floating calmly down the middle of the river.

Barriers to Feeling Better

LACK OF SAFETY

You cannot recover while you are still in the middle of trauma. First, you must get to safety. Otherwise, your nervous system will recognize that you still need your trauma responses, and they will continue.

Trauma may exist in a widespread sense in your community. This is particularly difficult if you are from a marginalized community and experience a lack of safety through racism, homophobia, or other forms of discrimination.

If you are trying to heal from trauma but cannot, it could be because you are not yet safe.

LACK OF SUPPORT

Traumatic experiences have a way of isolating you. Sometimes, this is due to the shame you may feel. Even though experiencing a traumatic event is not your fault, you may internalize it through a lens of self-blame—this can make it feel as though you had some kind of control instead of being completely helpless. But shame is isolating, and this isolation and the resulting lack of support tend to exacerbate the very shame that you are using isolation to try to escape.

You may be more vulnerable to PTSD and have more difficulty accessing care if you identify as a veteran, immigrant, or are living in poverty.[13] It may be helpful to utilize the support of your family, friends, and spiritual/faith community as you heal.

TRAUMA ACTIVATION (TRIGGERS)

You may find the term "trigger" to be distressing, especially if you have experienced gun violence. We use it here only as the common term that may help you when researching more about trauma. Trauma therapists tend to use the word "activation" instead, so we will do so throughout this book.

Despite your constant hard work to process your trauma in therapy and practice your coping skills, a trauma activation can sweep you right off your feet and sometimes feel like you go back all the way to your starting point.

"Activation" is the word we use when your nervous system experiences something reminiscent of your trauma. The activation itself can be something others think of as neutral or even positive, such as a scent, a song on the radio, or the weather. Because your brain has associated a seemingly innocuous stimulus with a dangerous situation, every time it experiences it again, it screams, "Danger!!" Activation can prevent you from enjoying things you used to love, and the destabilizing feeling of adrenaline, norepinephrine, and cortisol flooding your body can create your own personal horror movie even when things are actually quite safe.

This is a demoralizing and frustrating experience but know that when you are doing the hard work to recover from trauma, you are never truly back at the starting line. A better way to look at this can be like a spiral staircase: Sometimes it feels like you're going in circles, but with every step you are always making progress. Remember that every activating experience is just your brain and body responding to feeling unsafe exactly the way it's intended to. We can take a deep breath, feel our feet on the ground, and remind ourselves that we are in fact safe. Sometimes it is helpful to say aloud, "I am safe."

How To Communicate about Experiences with Trauma

IF YOU'RE THE ONE WHO EXPERIENCED TRAUMA

Know that you are not alone, and that while feelings of shame and self-blame may make it hard to reach out for support, it is important to do so.

Telling someone about your trauma history is a highly personal decision. It's important to feel confident that the loved one you are sharing with is a supportive person. You may say "I'm hoping to talk to you about a topic that's sensitive for me. Can we find a time and place where we both can feel safe?"

IF A LOVED ONE IS EXPERIENCING TRAUMA OR PTSD

Reach out, offer a listening ear, and most importantly, take a nonjudgmental stance. Know that your loved one may be judging themselves, and the last thing they need is to hear your ideas about how they could avoid future trauma or should have handled this experience differently. They simply need to know that you are there for them and that you care.

IF THE PERSON EXPERIENCING TRAUMA OR PTSD IS A CHILD

See chapter 7 for more about childhood trauma.

What Coping with Trauma and PTSD Can Look Like in Real Life

When Camila was a freshman in college, there was an active shooter on her campus. During the campus lockdown, she heard distressing noises and felt helpless and terrified. Camila survived the shooting without physical injury, and she thought she should feel grateful, but for the first few weeks she kept swinging back and forth between feeling numb and scared. When she felt numb, Camila would sleep all day and zone out during class. When she felt scared, she would be up all night, listening to every sound and wondering if she was safe. Camila also found herself feeling guilty for freezing during the shooting instead of rushing to help classmates. She ended up dropping out before the semester ended, hoping that she would feel safe back home.

However, Camila found that even at home she still had trouble sleeping, experienced numbness, and was easily startled. Her mom convinced her to try going back to school, but this time with the support of one of the campus therapists.

The therapist taught Camila that PTSD is a "biphasic disorder," meaning that it cycles back and forth between the phases of numbing and intrusive symptoms,[14] like how hypervigilant Camila sometimes felt at night (the intrusive phase) versus how she would zone out in class or sleep all day (the numbing phase). She found it helpful to think of these phases as the different zones she might encounter while floating down a river. Camila's therapist recommended that she connect with an EMDR therapist. Camila learned that through Adjunctive EMDR she could meet with a specialist for a brain-based therapy to change the way the memories of the shooting kept circulating through her mind.

Camila learned how to use deep breathing and grounding when she was on areas of campus that were particularly activating. After a few months of talk therapy and EMDR, Camila told her mom, "I can still remember everything that happened, but it feels far away now. Remembering doesn't set me back anymore." Camila also shared that one of the most important things she learned is that the freeze response is a completely normal part of a person's drive to survive.[15] Instead of feeling guilty for not being able to save her classmates, Camila learned to grieve their loss in a healthy way.

READING LIST AND OTHER RESOURCES

My Grandmother's Hands: Racialized Trauma and the Pathway to Mending Our Hearts and Bodies by Resmaa Menakem is a crucial read for anyone seeking to understand how trauma shapes our society, and the impact it's had on our bodies, especially the bodies of Black people in America. It also covers epigenetics and somatic healing.

The Body Keeps the Score by Bessel van der Kolk takes a clinical look at how trauma impacts the brain and the body. If you nerd out on science or need to understand the chemistry of what is happening to you or your loved one, this book is for you.

No Bad Parts: Healing Trauma and Restoring Wholeness with the Internal Family Systems Model by Richard Schwartz. If you feel you can't manage your trauma responses no matter what you try, it may be because parts of yourself are stuck in the trauma. This book by the founder of Internal Family Systems Therapy describes how each part works and how you can heal them.

The Living Legacy of Trauma Flip Chart by Janina Fisher is an educational resource to help you understand the impact of trauma on your body and your brain.

Tea With a Trauma Therapist (teawithatraumatherapist.com) is a course developed by Charity O'Reilly (one of this book's authors) to teach you about healing from trauma.

You can find more information about Trauma-Sensitive Yoga at traumasensitiveyoga.com.

KID-FRIENDLY TIP "Window of Tolerance Reimagined" is a YouTube video created by social worker Tracey Farrell. This animated short is great for both children and adults in describing trauma-related hyperarousal ("The Land of Fire") and hypoarousal ("The Land of Ice").[16]

For more resources, see the list on page 76.

7

DEVELOPMENTAL TRAUMA

You may not have heard the term "Developmental Trauma" before, but if you have experienced it, it's likely silently impacting your life every day. Some of the signs of Developmental Trauma include feeling a lack of trust or difficulty feeling safe with others and connected with yourself. You may often question why you have this difficulty, and try to motivate yourself to change, but something feels stuck inside you. You may say to yourself that your problems are "all in your head," but science tells us that's not true.

One of the first studies to make the link between Post-Traumatic Stress Disorder (PTSD) and our development in childhood was the Adverse Childhood Experiences (ACE) study. This study linked childhood trauma (ACEs) to negative adult medical outcomes, including addiction and early death, and was the foundation that developed understanding that, even when you do not meet the DSM (Diagnostic and Statistical Manual of Mental Disorders) criteria for PTSD, there are many types of life experiences that cause a similar trauma response.[1] This is often called Developmental Trauma, Attachment Trauma, or Complex PTSD (CPTSD).[2]

The ACE study found that children experiencing abuse (including physical, sexual, or emotional abuse), neglect (including emotional neglect and neglect due to poverty), witnessing domestic violence, having a family member who was mentally ill or incarcerated, having substance abuse in the household, or whose parents are divorced, are at an increased risk for strong negative outcomes. These include alcoholism and drug abuse, obesity, heart disease, cancer, and suicide attempts. The study "found a strong graded relationship between the breadth of exposure to abuse or household dysfunction during childhood and multiple risk factors for several of the leading causes of death in adults."[3]

According to the Children's Defense Fund 2023 report, 11 million children live in poverty in the US, "including 1 in 7 children of color and 1 in 6 children under 5."[4] Developmental Trauma is all too common in our society. Medical and mental health professionals agree that childhood trauma has "lasting detrimental impacts," and yet often remains underaddressed.[5] Childhood trauma affects brain development, including decreasing gray matter and increasing cortisol,[6] as well as other areas of functioning, which have a significant impact throughout the lifespan of the child.[7] If you are undergoing lasting impact from trauma you experienced many years ago, it's not "all in your head."

> **THE RESEARCH SAYS . . .**
>
> **You Are Not Alone**
>
> Sexual abuse is a childhood experience that creates Developmental Trauma. According to the National Center for Victims of Crime, one in every five girls experiences sexual abuse in childhood.[8] The statistics for boys may lag behind, but only because of underreporting, not because they are sexually abused less frequently[9] (see chapter 15).

What Professional Help May Look Like

PSYCHOEDUCATION

If you are working with a trauma-informed professional, one of the first things they will likely do is provide you with "psychoeducation," or information about how your Developmental Trauma has impacted you.

For example, children have long been called "resilient," and while this is true in some ways, as a blanket statement it creates the false impression that children are not impacted by events that they do not fully understand and perhaps will not remember. In fact, nothing could be further from the truth, as there are numerous factors that contribute to children being more significantly impacted from trauma the younger they are.[10] Often children are unable to make appropriate meaning or even any sense of their adverse childhood experiences, leaving them with a reactive nervous system they do not know how to calm.

Furthermore, because young children are completely dependent upon their caregivers, some of the hallmarks of trauma, including helplessness and intense fear, are most impactful for this age group.[11] Childhood trauma has far-reaching impacts that include a greatly increased risk for emotional suffering and suicide in adulthood.[12]

As you come to understand these dynamics through psychoeducation, you will be better able to offer yourself compassion for what you went through in childhood, and how it is impacting you now.

TRAUMA-INFORMED THERAPY

Eye Movement Desensitization and Reprocessing (EMDR), Trauma-Focused Cognitive Behavioral Therapy (TF-CBT), Internal Family Systems Therapy (IFS) and Trauma Sensitive Yoga (TSY) are some good examples of trauma-informed therapy models that may be useful to you as you heal from Developmental Trauma. See page 59 for more information on each of these therapies.

Trauma-informed therapy for Developmental Trauma is important both to free you from the impact of your childhood trauma, and to stop the transmission of intergenerational trauma, a process known as epigenetics.[13] If you are a parent with your own trauma history, one of the best things you can do for your child is work on your own trauma healing as proven by Dan Siegel's finding on parental healing being an important predictor of whether children will have a secure attachment style.[14]

Strategies to Try

TREAT YOURSELF WITH COMPASSION

Research has shown that PTSD symptoms actually decrease if you practice self-compassion.[15] Many survivors of childhood trauma find it difficult to do this, because of the internal messages they absorbed while their brains were still developing. Survivors of childhood sexual abuse may think things like *I am dirty* or *I am broken*. Survivors of childhood physical abuse may think things like *I have no control of my life*, or *I will never be safe*. When a child grows up believing these things, it takes real work to shift them.

Whether or not you plan to work with a therapist, you can challenge the distortions with new thoughts. It can be powerful to think of your younger self as you do this. Picture the younger you who went through that trauma; if you're comfortable doing so, look at a picture of you at that age. See if you can practice speaking to that version of you differently. Would you say, "You're broken!" to that child? Or would you perhaps say, "I am so sorry you went through that. It wasn't your fault." Keep having conversations with this younger part of you until you can offer this same compassion to yourself today, who is just a bigger version of that child. You can find more resources on how to work with your inner child in the Resources section of this chapter.

GET INVOLVED IN PREVENTING CHILD ABUSE

Survivors often ask for ways to get involved in helping ensure others don't have the same experiences. Whatever your role in society, if you are an adult, there are things you can do to protect children. Experts agree that adult understanding is necessary in reducing the epidemic of childhood exposure to trauma.[16] One such way is to attend community programs such as Darkness to Light's Stewards of Children Program or the Polaris Project's Human Trafficking Training.

Barriers to Feeling Better

CULTURAL NORMS

One of the reasons child abuse is so widespread is because of the cultural norms that protect it. For example, children are often taught and expected to do what adults request of them, no matter how they feel about it.

Many childhood sexual abuse survivors explain that their abuse began in seemingly innocuous ways, like being forced to hug or sit on the lap of an adult family member or friend who then gradually began abusing them, in a process known as grooming.[17] In a child sex offender's pattern of abuse, grooming enables them to keep children feeling connected to them, not scared and avoidant. Child abuse is able to continue because grooming behaviors, such as expecting children to be physically close to adults even if they don't want to be, are socially acceptable.

LACK OF SECURE ATTACHMENTS

Almost nothing impacts a child's chances of being resilient in the face of trauma more than their primary attachments.[18] Primary attachments are the caregivers that shape a child's world, first in utero, and then the people who are responsible for the child after birth. These are the people who make a child feel either safe or unsafe in the world from the moment they are born (or even before). If a child feels safe, they can go on to explore the world and begin to learn everything about it. If a child doesn't feel safe, these crucial developmental milestones will be hindered, missed, or experienced through a lens of helplessness and shame instead of confidence and hope. Not having secure childhood attachment will often mean a child does not have the resilience needed to cope with other childhood stressors, such as the ACEs discussed previously.

UNHEALTHY COPING STRATEGIES

If you have experienced childhood trauma, you've probably tried everything you can to cope. Often, these coping strategies become unhealthy over time.

Childhood trauma affects brain development, which has a significant impact throughout the lifespan of the child.[19] Those same children may develop a trauma response,[20] which they may attempt to cope with in ways that lead to further mental health and medical issues. For example, it is common for childhood trauma survivors to depend on using substances or food to cope with and numb their pain, which continues the cycle to the known medical and mental health outcomes from the ACE study, and possibly to the trauma cycle being carried into the next generation with their own children.

LACK OF COMMUNITY SUPPORT

Many children in the United States do not have access to the resources they need to grow into healthy adults (including environments that are physically safe, and adults who are emotionally safe), especially in the aftermath of trauma. Factors such as community violence, parents suffering from addiction, and poverty are widespread issues impacting the development of many children today. Marginalized communities often experience even fewer resources. For example, the public schools in Black and Brown communities often have less resources than those in white communities. Children who identify as LGBTQ+ often have fewer supports at home than children who don't—support that is critical to their development. This includes an enormous increase in youths who identify as LGBTQ+ becoming homeless, which leads to lack of access to basic life supports.[21]

How to Communicate About Developmental Trauma

IF YOU'RE THE ONE WHO EXPERIENCED CHILDHOOD TRAUMA

First of all, we want you to know that you are not exaggerating how bad your childhood trauma was and how much pain you sometimes feel because of it. As traumatized children grow into adults, it's typical for them to begin to minimize their experiences. This may be because it's what the adults in their world did. However, as the trauma symptoms persist, survivors of childhood trauma can begin to feel that there must be something wrong with them. Despite how difficult the healing process can be, there are numerous evidence-based supports available, and you deserve help and healing. The Resources section on page 66 will be helpful to you, too.

You may be unsure how much detail to share with your loved ones about your childhood experiences. This is a personal decision, and you can also ask your loved one what they are comfortable hearing. You may want to consider letting them know what kind of response would be helpful. Some people want to see how it impacts their loved one to hear their story, and others feel uncomfortable with this. What would feel safest and most supportive to you? If it feels too awkward, consider joining a support group first, to get some practice talking about your experiences in a supportive environment.

Consider sharing some of the science of trauma with your loved ones, either from this book or the books recommended in the Resources section in this chapter and on page 66. Many trauma therapists would be happy to have a joint session with you and your loved one so they can help you explain the very real impact of childhood trauma.

IF THE LOVED ONE WHO EXPERIENCED THIS IS NOW AN ADULT

You can normalize for them that their childhood experiences of trauma really do have lasting implications. It's not uncommon for adult survivors to feel like they should "be over it by now," even though the science is clear that this impact is significant and lasting. Your loved one may need to hear, "I'm sorry that happened to you. It was not okay to be treated like that as a child. Of course it's still impacting you," or, "Of course things have been hard as you try to recover from what happened in your childhood." "Of course," said with genuine compassion, can be the most powerful two words we can offer loved ones. If they are struggling from the impact, you can encourage them to seek trauma-specific treatment, especially EMDR or a trauma-focused version of CBT.[22]

IF THE LOVED ONE EXPERIENCING THIS IS STILL A CHILD

It's crucial to offer them age-appropriate support, and to connect them to professional intervention if needed. Children need to be reassured that the trauma is absolutely not their fault as their developmental stage may lead them to assume. They need to know they can talk to their support people about what happened to them when they want to, although they also should not be forced to talk before they are ready.

If you are a parent, your role is so important. A 2021 study found that "perceived parental care" was the only protective factor in helping sexually abused children avoid future traumatization, which means that parents play a pivotal role in their child's recovery.[23]

Children already feel helpless in so much of life, and it's important to not create more helplessness by forcing them to engage in support options they do not want to do. However, if professional intervention is needed, Trauma-Focused Cognitive Behavioral Therapy (TF-CBT; discussed on page 60) can be helpful.

Children often respond healthily to their experience of trauma; sometimes it's the reactions of their caregivers that cause the most stress and symptoms. So, for many traumatized children, it's just as important for their caregivers to go to therapy. Your mental health is a crucial part of your child's wellness! Plus, if you go to therapy it lets the child know that feelings and getting help for them are normal, and that there is nothing to be ashamed about.

If your child does not want to attend therapy, it's possible that they don't need to. Be open to that possibility. However, if it's clear that they do need extra support, ask them if they will attend a couple of sessions with the child trauma therapist and see what they think. Children often find they enjoy the experience when they meet with the right person.

What Coping with Developmental Trauma Can Look Like in Real Life

When Xander was born, their mother, who had her own history of childhood sexual abuse, was struggling with addiction and was unable to meet Xander's basic needs. Xander was assigned female at birth but knew from a young age that they did not identify as female. Their early experimentation with expressing their gender as nonbinary resulted in bullying and even being assaulted by a peer at school.

As a result of these traumas, Xander spent their young adulthood engaging in numerous codependent romantic relationships in an effort to find the security they were missing.

Because of their mom's addiction, Xander swore they would never use illegal drugs. However, they found different ways to numb themselves. When relationships didn't work, Xander would numb through self-injury. And sometimes they would feel numb for what seemed like no reason at all, a sensation like they were floating through life.

Xander finally found a stable relationship, but the self-harm had gotten to be a habit by then and their partner noticed. Their partner was upset by the self-harm and told Xander they needed therapy, so they sought support at their local sexual assault center. There, Xander met with a therapist who worked to help them understand that their symptoms were typical for someone who had experienced trauma since childhood.

The therapist called this "psychoeducation" and explained to Xander that when babies don't have their needs met, they can't securely attach to others or feel safe in the world, and instead develop one of three other attachment styles (avoidant, anxious, or disorganized) in order to try and find safety. Because of Xander's history of clinging to unhealthy relationships even when they were abusive, the therapist suggested that Xander may have developed an anxious attachment style.

The therapist also explained why Xander was numb, because when the brain is faced with unspeakable pain, like being sexually assaulted, it learns to shut down in order to protect itself. This is called dissociation, and the therapist shared how it is our brain's attempt to survive the trauma.

Xander agreed to engage in a form of trauma processing therapy called Eye Movement Desensitization and Reprocessing (EMDR) with their therapist. Using EMDR, Xander processed their traumatic memories going all the way back to childhood and working up through the bullying, assault, and abusive relationships. This was hard work, but their coping skills and their supportive partner helped them through it, and they saw their trauma symptoms reduce. Xander now says, "I know now that I was not a bad person because my mom couldn't care for me. I know I was doing the best I could to cope with all my trauma. I choose to see myself through the eyes of self-compassion, and it's making all the difference!"

READING LIST AND OTHER RESOURCES

What Happened to You: Conversations on Trauma, Resilience, and Healing by Oprah Winfrey and Bruce Perry explores many of the topics included in this chapter, including the ACE study and the impact of trauma on the developing brain, in an easy-to-read format.

The Tender Parts: A Guide to Healing from Trauma Through Internal Family Systems Therapy by Ilyse Kennedy is a reader-friendly guide to understanding your parts, with exercises to help you with the process.

It Didn't Start with You: How Inherited Family Trauma Shapes Who We Are and How to End the Cycle by Mark Wolynn guides you through epigenetics, or how trauma is passed down generationally, in a reader-friendly way.

The Myth of Normal: Trauma, Illness & Healing in a Toxic Culture by Gabor and Daniel Mate helps you understand the impact of trauma, in both a broad cultural and individual context.

Parenting from the Inside Out: How A Deeper Self-Understanding Can Help You Raise Children Who Thrive by Daniel J. Siegel and Mary Hartzell is a great resource if you are a parent with your own trauma history.

Polysecure: Attachment, Trauma and Consensual Nonmonogamy by Jessica Fern is an excellent resource for understanding attachment styles. While it is written for those who are in or considering a polyamorous relationship, the first half of the book is dedicated to helping you understand how your childhood attachment style impacts your adult relationships.

Reclaiming YOU: Using the Enneagram to Move from Trauma to Resilience by Sharon Ball and Renée Siegel helps you understand how to use the Enneagram to discover how your personality type is impacted by your trauma.

Nate Postlethwait has many resources on his website including a free e-book on healing trauma by connecting with your inner child: natewrites.com.

Darkness to Light's Stewards of Children Program (d2l.org/education/stewards-of-children) and the Polaris Project Human Trafficking Training (polarisproject.org/training) are educational programs that help adults learn about the issues of child abuse and the commercial sexual exploitation of children, so that they can become upstanders (instead of bystanders) in their community. You can find out more about both of these programs online.

For more resources, see the list on page 66.

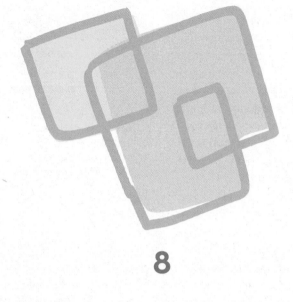

8

BORDERLINE PERSONALITY DISORDER

f you live with Borderline Personality Disorder (BPD), you have likely experienced challenging relationships and situations in your life. In many ways, BPD is a disorder marked by suffering. While research has not indicated a single cause for BPD, it has been linked to a history of childhood abuse and/or insecure attachment that creates emotional vulnerability,[1] and is widely thought to result from exposure to childhood trauma.[2] Because of this, clinicians who work with patients with BPD often find it helpful to classify it as a trauma disorder. If you have BPD, it is likely you are being affected by your trauma history, attachment difficulties, negative self-esteem, and mental or physical health.

The core of BPD is that you desperately want to have connections with others. Because of the trauma or lack of healthy attachments you experienced, you have not had an opportunity to develop healthy ways to nurture those connections or the connection with yourself. You may struggle with negative self-worth and assume that others are also thinking negatively of you. This may lead you to feel intense fear of being abandoned, although you may end up inadvertently pushing away the people you hope most to find support from, creating even more suffering. You may also engage in behaviors that others may see as manipulative in order to maintain relationships or get your needs met.

> **THE RESEARCH SAYS . . .**
>
> **You Are Not Alone**
>
> While only 1 to 2 percent of the general population is diagnosed with BPD, up to 22 percent of people in inpatient settings are diagnosed with BPD, demonstrating how unmanageable clinicians often feel it to be, leading them to recommend inpatient treatment more often than for other disorders.[4]

Managing your emotions can be challenging and you may try to cope through self-harm, such as cutting. Bottling up intense emotions inside you can spill over, sometimes in unhelpful, impulsive, and even destructive ways. You don't quite know how to respond to your emotions in ways that truly bring you connection and security. All of these challenges can create relational ruptures, long histories of mental health treatment or numerous inpatient hospitalizations, and suicide attempts.

Although BPD is one of the most common personality disorders, it is also among the most misunderstood conditions impacting mental and social health. It was previously believed that personality disorders wouldn't improve with therapy. This is far from the case. The struggles you experience due to BPD may be eased thanks to the advancements and advocacy of psychologist Dr. Marsha Linehan. Dr. Linehan developed Dialectical Behavior Therapy (DBT), the frontline treatment for BPD, and also has been a destigmatizing force for BPD, as she has shared her own journey living with the diagnosis.[3] Development of DBT and Dr. Linehan's efforts have moved us toward a more compassionate understanding of the realities of living with BPD and the best ways to empower yourself to live a full, healthy life.

What Professional Help May Look Like

Despite all of the stigma surrounding BPD and the impact this can have on treatment outcomes, you may experience relief upon receiving an accurate diagnosis of BPD.[5] It is important to note the emphasis on the word "accurate" here, as neurodiverse people, such as autistic people and those with PTSD, may be misdiagnosed with BPD.[6] However, when someone is accurately diagnosed with BPD, they may be able to access appropriate treatment for the first time.

DIALECTICAL BEHAVIORAL THERAPY

Dialectical Behavioral Therapy (DBT) is considered the frontline treatment for people with BPD.[7] In DBT, you learn skills to manage intense emotions, instead of detaching from painful feelings, and engage positively in relationships, which are often areas of struggle when living with BPD. You also learn radical acceptance, which is the skill of accepting the reality of a situation without getting lost in the "why me?" and knowing you can take steps to alleviate your suffering. Like many manualized treatments (step-by-step treatments that follow specific guidelines), DBT can run the risk of missing your suffering in favor of focusing only on symptom reduction. If you choose to seek DBT treatment, it's important to work with a clinician who understands you as a whole person and not as a collection of symptoms.

DBT will likely include both individual and group sessions. The group sessions are a crucial part of learning the skills needed to cope with the overwhelming emotions of BPD. Even if you don't like group settings, it's the best way to learn and practice DBT skills.

THE RESEARCH SAYS . . .

How BPD Can Impact Your Brain and Body

Similarly to people with Post-Traumatic Stress Disorder, people with BPD have the higher than average cortisol levels associated with people who have experienced chronic childhood stress.[8] In addition, both groups have decreased gray matter in their brains, which results in less cognitive flexibility and greater emotional instability than control groups.

BPD is linked to a vastly decreased life expectancy: twenty-two years less than the general population.[9] This may be a result of the physical health complications many people with BPD experience, such as diabetes and heart disease, and/or of the risk-taking behavior, including suicidality.

KETAMINE-ASSISTED THERAPY

Ketamine-Assisted Therapy may also be helpful.[10] Such treatment should always be supervised by a medical or mental health professional due to the associated risks.

Strategies to Try

REFRAME YOUR BPD AS YOUR BRAIN'S ATTEMPT TO MEET YOUR ATTACHMENT NEEDS

Recognizing exactly how your BPD shows up may be key both for you and the people you care about to understand your feelings. For example, many people refer to those with BPD as "manipulative," a term that serves to further stigmatize those with the diagnosis. Understanding BPD as a cluster of symptoms through which you are desperately trying to have your attachment needs met is a much more accurate way to view BPD, and results in more self-compassion.

PRACTICE PARTS WORK

Treating your BPD as a part of yourself, rather than your whole self, can be helpful as you work to experience a life of joy and wholeness. "Parts work," which can be found in many forms of therapy such as Internal Family Systems Therapy, as developed by Richard Schwartz, helps you identify the parts that have become burdened by trauma, and to learn to have compassion for them.

Considering your BPD as a part of yourself that is reacting to your trauma may give you enough space from your "BPD part" to decide how to help it. This could lead you to treat it with compassion, as well as understand that while it may try to run your life sometimes, it is not the whole you.

Barriers to Feeling Better

NEGATIVE SELF-CONCEPT

One difficult barrier to getting help comes from negative self-concept. A truism about BPD is that the things you accuse others of (such as thinking you are worthless or you're not worth the trouble) are often what you think about yourself.

If all of these hateful beliefs are actually a reflection of your own thoughts, it can be hard to summon the motivation to seek help. It can be difficult to even believe you deserve help. This contributes to feeling stuck in a vicious cycle.[11]

A VICTIM MINDSET

If you have BPD, it is true that you likely experience extreme suffering, both emotionally and even physically. It is likely true that your life circumstances have been painful and unfair. However, it is also true that no one is going to save you from your suffering except yourself. This is why the radical acceptance taught by DBT is often such an important part of the growth process.

THE IMPULSE TO PUSH LOVED ONES AWAY

Because of the intense emotional suffering and distorted view of self you may have, you may often push loved ones away, either verbally, through your behavior, or through self-sabotage. This not only exacerbates your feelings of abandonment and worthlessness, but it also distances you from the support that could be available to you. BPD is also considered an impulse control disorder,[12] making it difficult for you to restrain your impulses to push loved ones away.

STIGMA

If you have sought care for your BPD or other health struggles, you may have been faced with misunderstanding and negative assumptions. This is borne out in research, suggesting health care clinicians have more negative reactions to patients with BPD than patients with other mental health concerns, resulting in obstacles to effective caregiving.[13] This could lead you to feeling rejected, distrustful of the health system, and alienated in finding supportive care.

> **THE RESEARCH SAYS . . .**
>
> ### You May Also Experience These Things
>
> Because of the link between BPD and trauma, you may want to also check out chapters 6 and 7.
>
> If you live with BPD, you may also experience depression, anxiety, and chronic pain.[14] In short, BPD is an experience of extreme suffering, as indicated by the statistic that people who are diagnosed with the disorder are 45 percent more likely to attempt suicide.[15]

How to Communicate About BPD

IF YOU'RE THE ONE EXPERIENCING BPD

Whether or not you want to share the diagnosis is your decision, although people you want to connect with in healthy ways may benefit from understanding the symptoms and behaviors you experience.

If you know that you tend to have a hard time managing your emotions when you feel abandoned, you could say to loved ones, "Feeling abandoned, even if it's not true, is a big stressor for me. When things, like you forgetting we were going to hang out, happen, I might accuse you of not caring or say things to hurt you because I feel so hurt. I am working on this in therapy, but I want you to understand it's a current part of my relationship dynamics."

It's important to note that sharing this kind of information with loved ones is not an excuse to continue to hurt them. Rather, it's a way to stay honest and accountable when hurt occurs.

When your BPD symptoms do upset loved ones, it's important to respect their need for space or boundaries. You do not need to accept being intentionally hurt in return (which can happen in abusive relationships), but you do need to accept that a hurt person will need time and space to heal, and that they can choose if and when they are ready to continue connecting.

IF A LOVED ONE IS EXPERIENCING BPD

Having a healthy relationship with a person with BPD can be challenging, but it is possible. The most important factor determining this possibility is whether or not your loved one accepts that there are things they need to change. If they do not have this awareness, they will likely not be able to accept accountability for the harm they inadvertently cause in relationships. (See the "Stages of Change" section on page 105.)

Please do not "accuse" someone of having BPD. This is hurtful and leads to shame, not healing. If you think a loved one has BPD, focus on their symptoms, not the label. It is always best to do this by focusing on how their symptoms impact you. You could share that you feel overwhelmed by how they express their emotions and that you would like them to go to therapy to explore that.

The most important thing you can offer a loved one with BPD is consistency in your relationship. This means consistent support in whatever way you have space to offer it, and it also means consistent boundaries. Boundaries in relationships with a person with BPD provide safety for both of you to be yourselves and have your needs met. If you are struggling with boundaries in your relationship, it may be important to go to therapy to learn how to do this effectively. (We also address boundary setting on page 104.)

IF THE PERSON WITH BPD IS A CHILD

Clear communication and boundaries are an essential part of all relationships, but most especially in relationships with someone with BPD, as boundary violations caused by trauma are often a part of their lived experience. In fact, the research suggests that violations of parent/child boundaries are closely associated with the severity and persistence of BPD.[16] If your child has BPD, communicate household rules and expectations clearly, but without using control or guilt.

The crucial need to have firm boundaries without controlling a child perhaps demonstrates how important it is to seek professional guidance when it comes to BPD. If your child has BPD, both of you will likely benefit from a neutral third party who can guide you with expertise through the potential relational landmines.

What Coping with BPD Can Look Like in Real Life

Claire had always felt alone. When she was a child, she was often in "time out" for behaviors like temper tantrums and screaming "I hate you!" to her parents. Claire only wanted her parents to notice her—they were always so busy and as a result she felt invisible. She didn't have the words to express this and used the only means she knew—screaming and crying. Claire spent most of her time feeling like her emotions were going to make her explode because they felt so BIG, but she had no idea what to do about it except to just keep screaming.

As a teenager, Claire started finding new ways to manage her unbearable emotions, like cutting. After her mom saw the cuts on her thighs, Claire was put in therapy. From this, she realized that not only did cutting help her release the pain, but it made her feel seen, too. Claire vowed she'd never stop cutting. However, she wasn't honest about this with her therapist because she felt that they truly cared about her, and she didn't want to lose that connection. She also didn't want to lose the alone time with her mom in the car every week on the way to therapy.

After graduating, Claire got a job grooming dogs. Customers would sometimes see the scars on her arms, and Claire would tell them how much everything inside her hurt. Customers began to complain about Claire's oversharing, and she was soon fired. She felt that old rage building inside her in a way it hadn't since she'd started cutting. She stormed out of her manager's office screaming and pushed over an aquarium on her way out of the store. The police were called, and the next thing Claire knew, she had to go to court. The judge ordered that Claire go to a DBT group.

In the DBT group, Claire was taught a new skill every week on how to tolerate distress and manage her emotions instead of feeling as though they controlled her. It wasn't always easy, although she felt more empowered by being able to take a step back to breathe and think before she reacted. She also learned healthy ways to state her needs, and therapy sessions with her mom helped to strengthen their relationship. A moment of destruction led her to the beginning of her healing journey.

READING LIST AND OTHER RESOURCES

The Dialectical Behavior Therapy Skills Workbook: Practical DBT Exercises for Learning Mindfulness, Interpersonal Effectiveness, Emotion Regulation, and Distress Tolerance by Matthew McKay, Jeffery Wood, and Jeffery Brantley is an easy-to-use workbook that teaches many of the main components of DBT. You may find it helpful to go through the workbook with a therapist, or you may be comfortable using it on your own to practice DBT skills.

The Big Feelings Survival Guide: A Creative Workbook for Mental Health by Alyse Ruriani is a fun, colorful workbook that teaches DBT strategies in creative and accessible ways.

There are numerous books that address codependency and love addiction, which are sometimes side effects of BPD. These include *Facing Love Addiction: Giving Yourself the Power to Change the Way You Love*; *Facing Codependence: What It Is, Where It Comes from, How It Sabotages Our Lives* by Pia Mellody with Andrea Wells Miller and J. Keith Miller; *Codependent No More: How to Stop Controlling Others and Start Caring for Yourself*; and *The New Codependency: Help and Guidance for Today's Generation* by Melody Beattie.

You may find twelve-step groups for topics such as codependency (such as Co-Dependents Anonymous) or sex and love addiction (such as Sex and Love Addicts Anonymous) to be a helpful way to get support, even if you don't relate to those specific diagnoses.

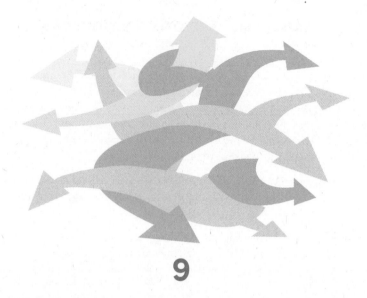

9

ATTENTION-DEFICIT/ HYPERACTIVITY DISORDER

Nowadays, it may seem your attention span is getting shorter and shorter. Our modern world, with access to social media and to deliveries to our front door in hours if not minutes, may make it feel harder to keep your attention on one task for long periods of time. While these struggles with attention are becoming more universal, it's important to recognize that this is *not* the same experience had by people with Attention-Deficit/Hyperactivity Disorder (ADHD).

ADHD is often considered to be an impairment of executive functioning, which encompasses working memory and time management,[1] as well as a type of neurodivergence. How this expresses itself is unique to you.

Although "impairments" are often used in clinical descriptions of ADHD, there are many gifts that a neurodivergent brain brings.

Some of the many strengths of ADHD and other neurodiverse conditions can include innovative thinking, strong attention to detail, hyperfocus, and creative, enthusiastic problem-solving.[2] You may report that these "super-powers" come into play especially when you are in novel situations, which may be linked to the novelty-seeking nature of ADHD connected to dopamine deficits in the brain.[3]

To be diagnosed with ADHD, you need to have a persistent pattern (at least six months) of six or more inattention and/or hyperactivity-impulsivity symptoms that interfere with your functioning or development.[4] You may have a combined presentation (meaning you experience both inattention and hyperactivity-impulsivity) or have predominantly inattentive or hyperactive-impulsive presentations, depending on the symptoms you experience. Here, you will find *some* examples of what you may experience if you have inattention or hyperactivity-impulsivity.

INATTENTION CHALLENGES

- You have trouble maintaining your attention during tasks, conversations, or during meetings/lectures.

- You have trouble paying close attention to details and may often make mistakes at work or school.

- You struggle with organization and may find time management near impossible. As a result, you may miss deadlines, and have heard comments from others about how "messy" your workspace is.

- You easily forget what you are doing, and may miss paying bills, making appointments, and completing and handing in assignments.

HYPERACTIVITY AND IMPULSIVITY CHALLENGES

- You may have a hard time sitting still, and often fidget in your seat.

- You may find that others have told you that you "talk too much" or too quickly.

- You may interrupt others mid-conversation because you feel an urgency to talk or may use someone else's things without asking.

- You are often "on the go" and others may describe you as having restless energy.

As someone with ADHD, you've experienced inattentive and/or hyperactivity/impulsivity symptoms that are present in multiple areas of your life; they have been present since before age twelve (even if you did not recognize it until adulthood); and they significantly impair your functioning in your relationships, work, and education, including in frequent changes of jobs, relationships, and residences.[5] If you were diagnosed with ADHD as a child, during adolescence your hyperactivity symptoms were more likely to have decreased while your inattentive symptoms remained stable.[6] You also may have experienced a full remission of your symptoms as you grew into an adult.[7]

If you have ADHD, reading that list may actually be difficult because of the challenges you experience with attention and focus. Many of the symptoms of ADHD would not be considered problematic outside of our traditional work and classroom settings. Words in the diagnostic criteria like "expected" and "inappropriate," and the rigidity of many environments, reveal just how much being neurotypical is baked into our perceptions of mental health. Because there is stigma associated with ADHD, many may "mask" their symptoms to blend in with social expectations, in which a person works to blend into the neurotypical world, often at great personal cost. Women especially are often not diagnosed until later in life due to their use of "masking."[8] As with other kinds of neurodivergence, oftentimes the problem is not you, but with society's expectations for you to fit within a neurotypical mold.

What Professional Help May Look Like

If you are seeking professional treatment for ADHD, it's important to work with a professional who respects neurodiversity. Your clinician should engage in shared decision-making by discussing treatment options with you. They will likely consider your age, the impact of the symptoms on your functioning, and other co-occurring diagnoses.[13]

MEDICATION

The frontline treatment for ADHD is medication. All medications have side effects, and it can take trials of many medications to find the best fit. This can be particularly challenging if you have ADHD, as you may find it difficult to follow through on tasks or appointments, including those connected to medication management.

ADHD medication, particularly stimulant treatment, has been shown to reduce the risk of mood disorders, suicidality, criminality, substance use disorders, accidents and injuries, educational underachievement, sexually transmitted infections, criminal activity, teenage pregnancy, traumatic brain injuries, motor vehicle crashes, and poor educational outcomes.[14]

Although stimulants are a frontline treatment for ADHD, they can come with concerning side effects, including anorexia, abdominal pain, headaches, sleep difficulties, and increases in blood pressure and pulse rate, and are also more likely to be diverted, misused, and abused.[15]

If you're looking for solutions outside of stimulants, you may find results with dopamine-related medications, such as bupropion.[16]

If you choose to use medication to treat your ADHD, it can be helpful to remind yourself that your medication is to assist your neurodiverse brain function in a system that was designed for a neurotypical brain. As always, speak with your clinician about what treatment may be the best fit for you.

COGNITIVE BEHAVIORAL THERAPY

There is some evidence that Cognitive Behavioral Therapy (CBT) may be beneficial for treating adults with ADHD, as a solo treatment or combined with medication.[17]

CBT for adults with ADHD includes a variety of strategies, such as organization, planning and time management skills, cognitive reappraisal strategies, and mindfulness meditation skills.[18] In general, CBT for ADHD should be thought of as a way to address the narratives that you may have acquired about yourself as a result of living in a neurotypical world (for example, feeling that you have to keep your ADHD a secret, or seeing yourself as lazy or an underachiever).

 ### PARENT-CHILD INTERACTION THERAPY

Parent training is recommended if you have a child or adolescent with ADHD or behavioral concerns that may be related to ADHD.[19] As with all concerns involving children, it is crucial for you or other family members to adapt and learn healthy behaviors as well. While not specifically designed for ADHD treatment, Parent-Child Interaction Therapy (PCIT) can help you learn how to interact with your child in the most effective ways, through live coaching with a PCIT therapist.

SPECIAL TREATMENT CONSIDERATIONS FOR CHILDREN AND ADOLESCENTS WITH ADHD

It is important to make sure your child is evaluated for ADHD and not to assume it because of normal behaviors such as having high energy. One Canadian study found that children born in December were 39 percent more likely to be diagnosed with ADHD, simply because they entered school in Canada as the youngest in their peer group.[20]

If you're concerned that your child may have ADHD, you can request a school evaluation. This can lead to accommodations and additional learning services to optimize academic performance.[21]

THE RESEARCH SAYS . . .

This Is How ADHD Can Impact Your Brain and Body

Brain imaging shows differences in the structure and functioning of the brain between people with and without ADHD,[22] including in the parts of the brain responsible for executive functioning.[23]

Researchers believe that there is a connection between ADHD and the dopamine and norepinephrine receptors in the brain, which is why some medications traditionally used to treat depression may be useful for treating ADHD.[24] This may also help explain the dopamine-seeking behaviors in which you may engage, such as excessive snacking, video game use, or risk-taking behaviors. Research is being targeted to develop treatments that will capitalize on this, such as game-based treatments.[25]

Genetics play a role in ADHD, and it is considered one of the most heritable mental health conditions, with a heritability rate of 76 percent.[26] This means chances are that if you have ADHD, other biological family members do, too.

While some caregivers struggle with the idea of their child being diagnosed, in many cases a diagnosis is the key to opening the door to both treatment and self-understanding.

It is often recommended that you receive a complete ADHD assessment, which includes a clinical interview, gathering information from loved ones and teachers, and testing such as intelligence tests and mood questionnaires.

If you are looking for someone who can provide this assessment for you, it is likely to be a psychologist or a therapist with specialized training in assessments. Check out chapter 24 to understand more about types of mental health clinicians.

Strategies to Try

GET ENOUGH SLEEP

If you have ADHD, you may also have difficulty with sleep.[27] A lack of sleep can make your ADHD symptoms worse.[28] If this describes you, see chapter 21.

REFRAME YOUR NEURODIVERSITY AS A "SUPERPOWER"

Your loved ones may become frustrated with you when it appears you don't hear them after they've made numerous attempts to get your attention, and that misunderstanding may lead you to feel depressed and anxious. You can alleviate the depression and anxiety associated with ADHD by reframing your neurodiversity as a "superpower" and practicing self-compassion. What appears to outsiders as inattention is often the hyperfocused ADHD brain at work. Rather than not being focused, it is unable to focus on extraneous tasks because it is so tuned in to the single task on its radar. Your "inattention" is not due to a lack of desire or willpower. Looking realistically at how your brain works and at its strengths can help you accept and cope with your diagnosis. Some examples of recognizing your superpowers are: "I have amazing attention to detail"; "I am a creative and outside the box thinker"; and "My energy brings a playfulness that lightens the room."

USE COREGULATION

Coregulation can mean a lot of things, but for neurodiverse people it typically means being present with another person (either in person or virtually) with whom you can adopt states of calm or focus. "Borrowing someone else's nervous system" is an idea from polyvagal theory and coregulation is a similar strategy that you can use to self-regulate.[29]

An important biological principle is that coregulation needs to come *before* self-regulation (for example, a newborn baby needing to sense calm from their caregiver before they can learn to self-soothe),[30] and for diagnoses such as ADHD that are hallmarked by emotional dysregulation, coregulation can be a meaningful tool.[31]

EXERCISE

Physical exercise, regardless of type, is helpful in targeting and reducing cognitive symptoms of ADHD, such as slow processing speed and distractibility.[32] You may feel much better when you regularly engage in physical exercise. Variety is also key for people with ADHD, so varying your exercise can help.

ASK FOR AND USE ACCOMMODATIONS

If you or your loved one are school-aged (this can include college) and diagnosed with ADHD, you can request accommodations, as ADHD qualifies as a disability in most schools. Such educational plans are made to optimize learning for children with disabilities, including extended test time, reduced homework, extra study materials, and supplemental class notes.[33]

While your workplace may not have set accommodations for people with ADHD, you may find that an honest conversation with your supervisor about useful supports (including coregulation through coworking, frequent check-ins about job performance from a positive reinforcement rather than punitive lens, and breaking big projects into smaller tasks) is helpful.

This is of course a case-by-case scenario dependent on your relationship with whomever you report to at work. If you do not report to anyone, putting such support structures into place with a coworker or ADHD coach can be helpful as well.

USE TO-DO LISTS

You may find it helpful to create to-do lists. Aim to keep the lists brief, no more than five tasks each time. Divide the lists by tasks that are to be completed that day and over the course of the week. If you find you are struggling with focusing on one task then switch to the next on your list. This can be helpful when completing tasks like chores or homework.

Be mindful to break down tasks that include multiple steps. If you write "complete project" on your to-do list for the morning and you know the project will likely take days to complete, then break it into smaller, more realistic, achievable tasks, and assign those to yourself over the course of multiple to-do lists.

Barriers to Feeling Better

SOCIETY'S POOR UNDERSTANDING OF NEURODIVERGENCE

The lack of understanding of neurodivergence can be frustrating. In its most basic definition, neurodiversity refers to the fact that not all brains function in the same way and resists defining a particular way that a brain with ADHD or autism operates as "good" or "bad," but simply as different or "diverse."

The neurodiversity movement has been helpful in allowing neurodiverse individuals to reframe their experiences. While the medical model can leave you feeling as though your diagnosis means there is something wrong with you, the neurodivergence approach lets you know that all the ways of functioning in the world are varied and valued.[34]

We encourage you and your loved ones to celebrate the ways your different approaches to thinking benefit the world. Both researchers and employers are beginning to realize that the differences of thought that neurodiversity brings are actually a bonus in the workplace.[35]

EXPENSIVE TREATMENTS NOT COVERED BY INSURANCE

Assessments and treatment for ADHD can be expensive and insurance may not always provide coverage.[36] Insurance may not even cover the cost of an assessment, especially for adults. This could result in needing to pay out of pocket, which can be prohibitively expensive.

When talking to your clinician, ask if they have low-cost recommendations in your community and call your insurance carrier to see if they offer coverage.

ADOLESCENCE

Adolescence can be a particularly tough time for someone coping with ADHD. Adolescents with ADHD are more likely to have lower levels of school attendance, more negative thoughts about their academic abilities, and lower self-efficacy. They engage in more negative social behaviors and are at a higher risk of self-harm.[37] If you know a teen experiencing ADHD, it may be a good idea to get them extra support, such as coaching, to help them navigate that time.

How to Communicate About Attention-Deficit/Hyperactivity Disorder

IF YOU'RE THE ONE WITH ADHD

Depending on your comfort level, tell others how they can best help you to stay on task and contribute. Let others know what proactive steps you're taking, and ask if they can help you utilize your strategies. Be mindful that others may periodically feel frustrated if they believe you are not contributing consistently in the way they may deem best, and that helping them understand the framework of neurodivergence may be useful.

Think creatively (often a strong suit of neurodiverse individuals!) about how you can contribute in ways that are meaningful and realistic for you. For example, tell others that you will be making a list, working on tasks in small concrete chunks, and that you plan to complete the overall goals, although it may take you a bit more time.

IF A LOVED ONE HAS ADHD

Patience and understanding is key. It may feel frustrating that they can play video games for hours (because video games reward the dopamine centers in the brain, making it easier to stay on task when dopamine is repeatedly released), but struggle to do the laundry (which most people would

---

THE RESEARCH SAYS . . .

You May Also Experience These Things

If you have ADHD, you may be more likely to have functional impairment (such as impairment related to employment and relationships) and higher rates of other mental health disorders.[38]

Most children diagnosed with ADHD also meet criteria for other behavioral health disorders, therefore the American Academy of Pediatrics recommends children and adolescents with ADHD be evaluated for mood disorders and past trauma (see page 67).[39]

If you are diagnosed with ADHD, you are at an "increased risk for obesity, asthma, allergies, diabetes mellitus, hypertension, sleep problems, psoriasis, epilepsy, sexually transmitted infections, abnormalities of the eye, immune disorders, and metabolic disorders." You are also at an "increased risk for low quality of life, substance use disorders, accidental injuries, educational underachievement, unemployment, gambling, teenage pregnancy, difficulties socializing, delinquency, suicide, and premature death."[40]

agree doesn't exactly release dopamine). Have clear and detailed conversations about how you feel and how you are hoping they can contribute. Remember that your loved one's inattention is part of their diagnosis and is not intentional. When possible, offer coworking/coregulation as a supportive strategy. Sometimes suggesting simple strategies (sharing physical space to accomplish tasks, making lists, breaking goals into small steps) is the most helpful approach.

IF THE PERSON WITH ADHD IS A CHILD

We understand that the decision to pursue a diagnosis is a complicated one, and the decision to provide medication to a child is more complicated still. We cannot presume to know your individual situation. However, we know from the research that untreated childhood ADHD can lead to significant negative adult outcomes, including in education, work, relationships, and risk-taking behaviors.[41]

Consider collaborating with your child on their ADHD diagnosis and treatment. They are likely very intelligent, even if it is expressed in different ways. Help them to see their ADHD skills as superpowers, and also to recognize their limitations and ways in which they may need additional support. Make the type of support you offer an ongoing dialogue with your child, who is likely to be an out of the box, creative thinker.

What Coping with Attention-Deficit/ Hyperactivity Disorder Can Look Like in Real Life

Nate started his freshman year of college two months ago, and it's been rough. He got Cs and one D on his midterms. He reviewed the material and thought he'd do okay, but when test-time came, he found it almost impossible to focus. No matter how many times he read the questions, he just couldn't make sense of them. He even ran out of time on one of the exams, which never happened to him before.

Nate was a straight-A student in grade school and high school. He barely needed to study and he could goof off in class and still get good grades. Sure, he'd sometimes forget assignments or procrastinate on projects until the last minute, but he was always able to make up the work or get extra credit. His teachers would say, "You're so smart—if only you applied yourself!"

Nate struggled socially, because it was hard for him to read social cues. Teachers complained to his parents about him talking with his friends during class and getting out of his seat without permission, but it never seemed to create problems for him because he got such good grades.

He asks one of his professors how he could improve his grade. Nate explains to them how good his academics had been in the past, and they encourage him to go to the school counseling center to ask about having an assessment completed.

Nate meets with a psychologist for two testing sessions that last several hours each. After a few weeks, he meets with them to hear the outcome and they tell him that he appears to meet criteria for ADHD.

Suddenly, Nate's current inattention and trouble focusing and his rambunctious activity as a child make a bit more sense. The psychologist shares with Nate that his IQ is in the above average range and so he was able to find strategies to help him perform well in school growing up. However, college has less structure and much more dense and complicated material to learn, so his old strategies aren't working.

With this diagnosis, Nate qualifies for accommodations. He is able to get extra time to complete exams. He also talks with his primary care clinician about possibly starting a medication. He attends appointments at his college counseling center to review mindfulness, Cognitive Behavioral Therapy, and study strategies, and he finds a study buddy to help him coregulate. After joining an online forum for people with ADHD, he learns about how ADHD is considered a neurodiversity. This understanding helps him reframe his diagnosis as a strength, which helps him through the bouts of depression and anxiety that sometimes come.

READING LIST AND OTHER RESOURCES

Laziness Does Not Exist by Devon Price challenges the social construct of "laziness" and shares reframing strategies that people, especially neurodiverse/ADHD people, may find helpful.

ADHD for Smart Ass Women: How to Fall in Love with Your Neurodivergent Brain by Tracy Otsuka is a book that helps women understand how ADHD may impact them, especially since it is often different from the male-focused depictions of ADHD most people are familiar with.

Unmasking Autism by Devon Price explores many of the nuances of neurodiversity, including ADHD.

Focusmate is an online resource that can help with coregulation. It connects you with another person looking to co-work or coregulate for a specific time span, such as an hour. Using a virtual platform, both users can complete their tasks with the benefits of coregulation. Focusmate is free for limited periods of time, or you can subscribe for unlimited sessions.

Habitica is an app that turns life tasks, like doing chores or taking medication, into a game with rewards. This is particularly helpful if you need dopamine to help you complete tasks.

You may find normalization and new coping strategies in online communities. Reddit.com/r/ADHDwomen is a frequently shared source, although as with all online recommendations, we cannot vouch for everything that will be shared.

The podcast *Search Engine* by P. J. Vogt has a two-part episode about the pros and cons of stimulant medication for ADHD called "Why'd I Take Speed for 20 Years?," which first aired in November 2023.

2

SOCIAL HEALTH

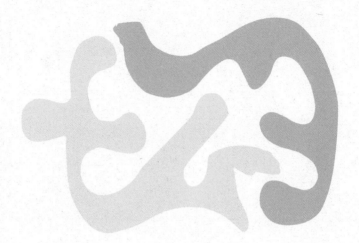

10

INTERPERSONAL RELATIONSHIPS

S ometimes healthy relationships can feel impossible to achieve. Often, this is because early in life, you developed a "template" of what a relationship looks like, based on your early childhood attachments (see also chapter 7).

If you had exposure to healthy communication early on, you may have felt safe to share your feelings knowing that your needs would be met. However, if you didn't have that sense of security, you may have found yourself "walking on eggshells" in order to avoid upsetting a family member. These experiences may have led you to learn that relationships are unstable, unsafe, and one-sided, which doesn't have to be the case.

Instability and lack of security in your environment and core relationships as a child can impact how you navigate relationships as an adult. If healthy boundaries weren't practiced, you may have a challenging time setting and maintaining appropriate boundaries for yourself. You may find yourself more in a people-pleasing role, in which you ignore or may not even recognize your wants and needs, in order to avoid conflict and maintain the status quo. You may shut off the desire for healthy relationships in order to protect yourself from being heartbroken if they don't work out.

THE RESEARCH SAYS . . .

This Is What's Happening in Your Brain and Body

A twenty-second hug with a loved one can lead to lowered heart rate and blood pressure.[5] If that feels uncomfortable, you can use the containment hug, where you put your left hand under your right armpit and right hand on your left shoulder, to mimic a hug.

You may also experience codependency within your relationships, where you lose your sense of self as you tend to the needs of others.[1] This may leave you feeling as though your worth is dependent on another person, and without that person, you feel lost and without purpose.

Positive social relationships are essential to your mental and physical health—and unhealthy relationships have a slew of negative impacts.[2] In this chapter, we will explore ways to improve relationships, although it is important to note that not all relationships can be improved, especially if there is abuse or fundamental incompatibility.

What Professional Help May Look Like

EMOTIONALLY FOCUSED THERAPY
Emotionally Focused Therapy helps individuals and couples build emotional regulation skills and explore their attachment styles to create safe emotional connections to both reduce and better manage conflict.[3]

ATTACHMENT-BASED FAMILY THERAPY
Attachment-Based Family Therapy involves working with the family unit to repair attachment wounds,[4] a crucial part of healthy relationships.

10

INTERPERSONAL RELATIONSHIPS

UNDERSTAND YOUR RELATIONSHIP DYNAMICS

It's important to take time to reflect on what has contributed to your perceptions of how relationships "should" be and what having a healthy relationship means to you.

Here are some journal prompts to help you explore this.

- What role do you take within relationships?
- Do you feel safe to share your wants and needs?
- Does it feel challenging to identify your wants and needs?
- Do you identify as a people pleaser?
- Do you withdraw during an argument? Or do you use your words as weapons?
- What is your relationship with vulnerability?
- What models have been set for you in what a relationship looks like?
- What was communication like in your household growing up?
- What helps you feel secure and safe in a relationship?
- What do you consider to be a healthy relationship?
- Does the idea of being in a healthy relationship feel foreign and unfamiliar?
- What does your relationship with yourself look like?

REPAIR YOUR ATTACHMENTS

Attachment repair means that while ruptures (fights, misunderstandings, or any other disruption in secure attachment) are inevitable in relationships, repair is what is most important. Even when a relationship is on rocky ground, if both people are willing, repair is possible.

Acknowledge the reality of what happened. Attachment repair cannot happen as long as either party is denying that a rupture happened. Being honest about the hurt is the first part of healing it. That may look like, "I lashed out at you, and it was not your fault."

Validate the other person's reactions. You don't have to excuse bad behavior but being able to understand how the other person feels through empathy is a nonnegotiable part of attachment repair.

Own your role in the rupture. In twelve-step groups, this is known as "keeping your side of the street clean." It's easy to focus on what the other person did wrong, but how did you contribute to the rupture? This is why it's important to start by acknowledging what happened and validating the hurt, because once you are experiencing compassion for the other person, it's much easier to own your part.

Offer repair. This looks different in every situation. Sometimes it looks like a genuine apology (not an apology trying to fast-forward through the hard parts) or making amends in some way. Other times, it looks like spending quality time together or sharing gratitude for each other. Ask the other person what repair would look like for them. Answer this question for yourself, situation by situation, too.

PRACTICE GRATITUDE

You may focus on what could go wrong in your relationships, instead of what has gone right. Practicing gratitude changes this.

Take a moment each day to identify one quality or action that you're grateful you performed today. Then share with a loved one something about them that you are grateful for or why you are grateful that they are in your life.

 If you have kids, try practicing gratitude as a family. This could look like sharing what you're grateful for at mealtimes or bedtime, or starting a family gratitude jar. Teach your children (and by extension, yourself) that gratitude is not about forcing a positive outlook but being aware of both the good and the hard things in life, choosing to notice them both and to savor the good.

CHECK IN WITH YOUR LOVED ONES

Take five minutes, however many days a week that feels right for you, to check in with your loved ones about how they are doing, what has been a highlight or lowlight of their day, and what they may need in terms of support. Model what you want to receive. If you want to hear real vulnerability, make sure you are sharing that yourself.

 Some families call this "pits and peaks" or "roses and thorns" and choose to do it around the dinner table or at another set time.

SET BOUNDARIES

Boundaries are about making clear how you want to be treated by others and are essential in healthy relationships. Think of a boundary as a fence around your well-being. You can't stop someone from trying to climb over your fence, but by putting the fence up, you are communicating your needs and desires. As uncomfortable it may feel to set and maintain boundaries, you are allowed to do so. Keep in mind that a true boundary is a kindness to you and everyone around you, so that everyone knows what to expect. As the author Brené Brown says, "Clear Is Kind."

Boundaries can be small or big declarations. It may be protecting your self-care time by not responding to a text immediately, or saying, "I'm sorry, I already have plans," to protect your peace. Small boundaries give us the space we need to set the bigger ones.

You may think of self-care as luxurious acts, like taking a vacation or having a spa day, but really those things are self-comfort. True self-care means doing difficult tasks that make our lives healthier overall, like exercising or going to therapy. Setting a boundary is self-care, because it's not about saying no to others; it's saying yes to yourself and what is healthiest for your life.

Sometimes the most important boundaries to set are with the people we love most, but who also drain our energy. Boundaries invite others to treat you in ways that will make it possible to remain in a relationship with them and are therefore an act of relational love.

In some circumstances, setting boundaries may not feel safe. We encourage you to utilize your support system so that you may move forward in a way that will be best for you.

EXPLORE YOUR VALUES

Do you know what you find important in your relationships? What helps you feel safe and supported? A great way to find out is through a values exercise. Think of five to ten values that you want present in your friendships, romantic relationship(s), and with your coworkers, and write those down.

If you are struggling to come up with some values, reflect on relationships that didn't feel healthy. You may find what you value is the opposite of what you experienced. If you felt invalidated, maybe the value of support or communication was missing. If you felt lonely, possibly the values of emotional intimacy and trust weren't there.

After you decide on your values, define what they mean to YOU. How do you know that your values are being met if you can't relate to them being present at all? If you choose 'respect' as one of your values, what would it look like to be treated with respect, or for you to treat someone else with respect?

Consider sharing these values with a loved one and ask them if they'd do the same. Discussing your values is a great way to see if they are shared, and to see if there are any needs that are not being met.

CULTIVATE YOUR RELATIONSHIP WITH YOURSELF

One of the relationships we often forget to nourish is the one we have with ourselves. How do you treat yourself? Mentally? Emotionally? Physically? When you take care of yourself, you are also able to show up for others in a way that's healthy for you. Doing the values exercise above may make it easier for you to know what you value for yourself.

Boundaries and self-care ultimately make us more able to have healthy relationships. Make sure to keep your cup of emotional, mental, physical, and spiritual health full.

Barriers to Healthy Relationships

BEING IN DIFFERENT STAGES OF CHANGE

Establishing a healthy relationship requires both you and your loved one to make changes. If you're not aligned in your openness or ability to make the necessary changes, it can present a challenge. "Stages of change" is a model used by therapists to evaluate your readiness to make change.[6] When it comes to relationships, it's important to recognize that you can't coerce someone to move from one stage to the next, but you can support them where they are.[7] People cycle in and out through the phases instead of proceeding in a linear fashion.[8]

Precontemplation is the stage of change when you are not yet aware that change needs to be made. This can look like "blissful ignorance," although considerable damage can still be happening behind the scenes, like when the roof of your house is leaking but you haven't noticed yet.

Contemplation is when you are aware that change is necessary, but you have not taken steps toward it. Others may feel frustrated with you because of your lack of action.

Preparation is when movement starts to happen. You may begin talking to others about the problem, reading or even going to therapy about it, and are thinking of the best approach to tackle it. This stage can feel frustrating for those around you, as there is understanding but no change happening yet.

Action is the stage when you take steps to be different. Perhaps you start communicating honestly, or engaging with how the other person feels. However, this may be a point when attachment ruptures occur.

One kind of rupture happens because you are taking action, but there are missteps. This can be a high-conflict time as you try to work out the details of what real behavior change looks like. Another common kind of rupture is due to what therapists call "the relational dance." All relationships are dances, in a way. You know your steps and your partner knows theirs. But when true behavioral change starts to happen, your new dance steps will require your partner to change theirs, too. This may be upsetting or even scary, and you'll need to persevere through it with openness and honesty.

Maintenance is the final stage where you are continuing to take active steps and give resources not only to the positive change, but to prevent engaging in old patterns. Maintenance may be where you can finally take a deep breath and relax into this new relational "dance," but like anything in life, relationships take ongoing work.

Like the house with the leaky roof, it's important to stay aware of and take proactive steps toward maintaining healthy relationships. Undoubtedly you and your partner will soon find a new relational change to make. If that's the case, you're doing relationships right!

POOR SELF-WORTH

If you don't think highly of yourself, you may also find that you are or have been in relationships in which you felt invalidated, taken advantage of, and not supported. You may also struggle with setting boundaries, stating what you want or need, and walking away from toxic relationships.

Poor self-worth can also involve shame. Shame is a relational template that is often set for us early in life. When children encounter trauma, especially attachment wounding, they aren't in a position to blame the grown-ups for what is happening, because they depend on those same grown-ups for their survival. Instead, they blame themselves. This becomes internalized as shame. Shame keeps us from healthy relationships because, instead of seeing things as they truly are, which means both taking healthy responsibility for our stuff and letting others take responsibility for theirs, we take on all the responsibility and end up in codependent relationships.

LACKING A MODEL FOR HEALTHY RELATIONSHIPS

If you haven't had a healthy model for relationships, you may find it more challenging to both recognize what is healthy and to navigate being in a healthy relationship. You may even feel uncomfortable in the unfamiliar stability of a healthy relationship. This may lead to pushing your partner away, engaging in unhealthy coping behaviors, or having trouble accepting the healthy and supportive love you truly deserve.

If this describes you, consider processing your past attachment trauma in order to find the freedom to give and receive in a healthy relationship. If you can't model your relationship on a parent or other family member, try modeling it on someone else you know, or even someone fictional. You can think about TV or book characters when you are imagining how to have a healthy relationship.

MISUNDERSTANDING NEURODIVERSITY

In relationships, the different ways the human brain functions can sometimes be seen as being problematic, when in reality they should be celebrated.

Autism is one form of neurodiversity that can be misunderstood in relationships. If you are autistic, you may feel overstimulated by new situations or loud places, which define many social settings. You may think in ways that are completely logical and yet are different from the way an allistic (non-autistic) person thinks, making it harder to communicate. But when allistic and autistic people learn to understand and appreciate their differences, relationships can be even stronger as a result. Be curious about others' experiences, ask questions, and imagine what it may be like to be them.

LACK OF RECIPROCITY

If the relationship you're in depends on you always giving more or you feel that you can't assert your wants and needs, you may want to consider how healthy it is for you. There needs to be reciprocity in relationships. We may not always be able to give the same amount all the time, but it's important that there is an overall balance of giving and taking.

There are times that no matter how much you change and grow, a relationship is not going to work. Giving yourself permission to walk away when needed is sometimes the best thing you can do for both you and the other person.

REFUSING TO TAKE RESPONSIBILITY

Sometimes the problem in the relationship is that you don't see or take responsibility for the issues you are causing.

If you think this may be you: Congratulations on recognizing it! It can be hard for people to see this dynamic in themselves.

Recognizing it is the first step, and the next is to take accountability.

Maybe you don't actually see this in yourself, but your loved ones keep saying it's true. What would happen if you experiment with the possibility of making changes in response to what your loved ones have shared? If your relationship improves, that may be the evidence you need that you weren't keeping your side of the street clean.

TOXIC DYNAMICS

Continuous rupture, in which repair is not coming from all parties or is not possible, is likely a sign of abuse, narcissism, or other conditions in which it is unfeasible for a relationship to thrive. Repair between adults should be a two-way process. If you are continuously offering repair but the other person is not engaging with it in responsible ways, it is possible that this relationship is not healthy or safe.

It is also possible that this is due to your own attachment patterns. If you are the one who cannot participate in attachment repair, it may be time to seek Trauma-Informed Therapy so that you can heal your past patterns and be open to new ones.

How to Communicate in Your Relationships

IF YOU'RE THE ONE STRUGGLING WITH YOUR RELATIONSHIPS

Consider "I" statements when communicating your feelings to others. Let your loved one know that you are practicing "I" statements and that you may need some extra support in this process.

"I" statements help us to identify our feelings in response to what is or isn't occurring within a relationship. It can also diffuse the accusatory statements that lead people to feel defensive, for example, "I feel disrespected and not valued when you don't follow-through" rather than "You make me feel horrible." It can also be helpful to use "we" language along with "I" statements. For example, "I feel sad when we are not able to spend time together. Could we look at our schedules to see what works for both of us?"

One challenge in communication is that you can present your thoughts and feelings in a loving and respectful way, yet the other individual may react from their own insecurities, which may not always result in the outcome you hoped for.

Healthy communication takes time to build, and investment from both parties. Going to couples or family therapy can be helpful in having someone walk you through healthy ways to navigate conflict and build trust and communication.

If all involved in the relationship work to respect each other, listen openly, and put love before ego, the result can be increased trust and security.

IF A LOVED ONE IS STRUGGLING WITH A RELATIONSHIP

Consider asking them the following questions.

- How can I support you in maintaining the boundaries you set? Do you want me to check in to see if you feel that you're honoring your boundaries?

- What do you want from the relationship?

- How do you feel you are being treated in the relationship?

- Do you feel that you are respecting yourself?

IF THE PERSON STRUGGLING WITH A RELATIONSHIP IS A CHILD

Modeling is key. Modeling trust, boundaries, healthy communication, and attachment repair with both them and others is how your child will learn what healthy relationships are.

Start small. Don't expect yourself to be the perfect parent (no one is!), but instead challenge yourself to work on one healthy relationship task with your child until it becomes the new normal, and then pick another and start again. You could practice "I" statements or sharing gratitude with each other.

Aim for about twenty minutes a day of unconditional time to spend with your child doing whatever they want, such as coloring, playing a game, engaging in imaginative play, or just talking about the day. The activity itself isn't important (although it can't be an activity you require of your child, such as homework). Unconditional time should happen daily, no matter what. It creates secure attachment, so your child knows they are safe and loved, which is the greatest gift you can give them.

What Building Healthier Relationships Can Look Like in Real Life

Charlotte grew up in a household where there was constant arguing. Sometimes the arguing would go from yelling to the silent treatment. The silent treatment felt worse, because at least when someone was yelling at her, Charlotte felt like she was acknowledged. Arguments were never resolved; everyone acted like everything was okay. It was exhausting, and she remembers always feeling on edge.

As a result, Charlotte would try desperately to keep the peace. To keep her parents happy, she wouldn't say what she wanted or needed. Sometimes, she'd get validated for it. Her parents would say, "You're such a good kid. You never cause any trouble." She took that to heart: If you don't cause any trouble, then you're good . . . and you're wanted. She carried that belief into her adult relationships.

She's been in a romantic relationship for about a year now. The partner she's with is kind and supportive. Occasionally, they disagree, and when that happens, Charlotte feels deeply uncomfortable. Since she was a kid, disagreements led her to shut down and she would do everything she could to make the conflict go away as quickly as possible. She's lived so much of her life being the peacemaker that she's terrified of potentially creating waves.

Charlotte's tendency to not consider herself and focus on her partner is putting a strain on her relationship. This is the first time she's experiencing this; a partner who wants her to focus on taking care of herself and to voice her needs. It feels so foreign. She's only been with partners who want to take, and her wants and needs were never prioritized.

She thinks to herself, *Okay, I have some stuff to work out*, and connects with a therapist. She learns skills to help regulate her emotions, particularly when she feels as though someone is not happy with her or when a disagreement is occurring.

Charlotte leans into identifying and saying what she needs, and her partner supports her. She begins to feel more secure within her romantic relationship, but even more importantly, she feels more secure within herself. In that security, she sets boundaries, with herself and for herself. Setting boundaries with her parents is difficult. It's like she's a little kid all over again, although she is showing her inner child that it is okay to stand strong when it comes to what is healthy for her.

READING LIST AND OTHER RESOURCES

Becky Kennedy explains attachment parenting in her book *Good Inside: A Practical Guide to Becoming the Parent You Want to Be*. It teaches parents how to see the good in their children, and her website offers a wealth of information including workshops. You may also enjoy her interviews in episodes 130, 131, 169, 170, and 267 of Glennon Doyle's podcast *We Can Do Hard Things*.

Hold Me Tight: Your Guide to the Most Successful Approach to Building Loving Relationships by Sue Johnson uses the Emotionally Focused Therapy framework to guide you through discussions about how you may approach relationships and engage in communication, and how your attachment style plays a primary role in how you relate to the world.

The Gifts of Imperfection by Brené Brown is a great book if you are looking to delve into a deeper relationship with yourself. Her book *Atlas of the Heart*, which has also been made into a five-part docuseries, may also help you understand your emotions better. And one of our most-recommended resources of all time is her talk "The Power of Vulnerability," which you can buy as an audiobook.

Facing Codependence: What It Is, Where It Comes from, How It Sabotages Our Lives by Pia Mellody with Andrea Wells Miller and J. Keith Miller explores the childhood experiences that may shape codependency in adulthood and discusses how to reach healing.

Codependent No More: How to Stop Controlling Others and Start Caring for Yourself and *The New Codependency: Help and Guidance for Today's Generation* are two books by the pioneer of discussing codependency, Melody Beattie. If you'd rather listen to a podcast, you can check out interviews with Melody Beattie, including episode 142 of Glennon Doyle's podcast *We Can Do Hard Things*, or the November 22, 2023, episode of Jen Hatmaker's podcast *For the Love*.

The Human Magnet Syndrome: Why We Love People Who Hurt Us by Ross Rosenberg explores why you may find yourself in relationships with partners who ultimately hurt you.

Sometimes everything is going well in your relationship, but you are struggling with intimacy. *Better Sex Through Mindfulness: How Women Can Cultivate Desire* by Lori Brotto and *Come as You Are: The Surprising New Science that Will Transform Your Sex Life* by Emily Nagoski are excellent books that can help you reconnect sexually with yourself and your partner. *Pillow Talks* is a podcast by sex therapist Vanessa Marin and her husband that walks you through many questions about sex—even the ones you didn't know you had!

The Gottman Institute (gottman.com) has several resources, some free and some paid, for couples and parents working to build healthy relationships, and improve communication.

For parents looking to navigate their new relationships with their toddlers, the online community Big Little Feelings (biglittlefeelings.com) provides support, insight, and a nonjudgmental approach.

You may find using personality typology helps you understand yourself and relate to others better. The Enneagram is a typology that focuses on motivations and childhood wounding instead of behavior. You can find free or paid versions of the Enneagram test online, but don't just take the test and assume it's true. Use the results to research more until you've found your type, and then use the understanding to deepen your relationships.

There are also many Enneagram coaches and workshops available online. You could consider Kaleigh Newby for using the Enneagram to improve romantic and work relationships, and Elisabeth Bennett from Enneagram Life who works from a faith-based perspective.

Adult Children of Alcoholics & Dysfunctional Families, previously known as Adult Children of Alcoholics (ACOA), is an organization that provides a twelve-step program for adults who grew up in households where they experienced abuse, neglect, and trauma. Find a local group at adultchildren.org.

Where Should We Begin? with Esther Perel, a renowned couples therapist, is a weekly podcast inviting people to listen in to couples' sessions with her. She has also released a board game of the same name that helps people connect through conversations.

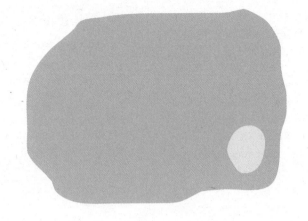

11

LONELINESS

eeling genuine social connections is integral to your overall health and well-being. Those connections provide you with a sense of belonging, letting you know that you're cared for, heard, and seen. Lacking meaningful social connections can lead to increased risk of premature death; that risk is the same as if you were smoking up to fifteen cigarettes a day.[1]

Loneliness is described as feeling emotional distress regarding your social needs not being satisfied, and the experience of perceived or actual isolation.[2] Social isolation is having little to no social interactions and may result from intrapersonal (such as self-talk or self-perception), behavioral, or environmental factors.[3] This doesn't necessarily mean that if you isolate (or are alone) that you also feel lonely. You may intentionally isolate and find it rejuvenating, or even preferred. Similarly, you can be surrounded by people and feel profound loneliness.

Quality relationships, meaningful daily interactions, and low social anxiety serve as protective factors in not experiencing loneliness and the impact of it.[4] However, while multiple avenues for connection are available today, the rate in which we experience loneliness has only increased, and significantly worsened during the height of the COVID-19 pandemic. As a result, loneliness has been deemed a public health concern that is occurring not only in the US, but in a significant portion of the world.[5]

Strategies to Try

CONNECT WITH YOUR COMMUNITY

Our communities are rich in social resources. Joining your local newspaper, church, library, animal shelter, community center, or your community/neighborhood/city's social media may provide you with a calendar of events to take part in.

Free local social activities may include a local library book club, groups for local politics, moms of preschoolers, church, meet-ups, community enhancement or gardening, and twelve-steps.

WORK TO STRENGTHEN YOUR EXISTING RELATIONSHIPS

If you have an old friend, chances are you were friends for a reason and could still find a connection point. Even if you haven't talked in a while, if they're someone you truly enjoyed sharing time with, make that call, schedule that lunch, and be present.

INVEST IN QUALITY CONNECTIONS OVER QUANTITY OF CONNECTIONS

Invest time in relationships that help you feel validated and valued for who you are. You want connections with others that you truly trust, feel safe with, and can rely on.

If you feel lonely even though you have plenty of relationships, consider evaluating which of them are two-way streets that bring you joy, and which of them are depleting you. (Also check out chapter 10, and in particular the codependency resources listed on page 85.)

CULTIVATE YOUR RELATIONSHIP WITH YOURSELF

One of the relationships we often neglect to nourish is the one we have with ourselves. What is the dialogue running through your mind? Are you being kind to yourself? Thinking about what you truly need? Make efforts to challenge your negative self-talk and reflect on why you may feel lonely in your own company.

In many senses, you are never alone because you always have yourself. Yes, having meaningful relationships with others is important, but remember that you take yourself everywhere.

CONNECT WITH ANIMALS

Bonding with animals can be therapeutic. Most local SPCAs offer opportunities to foster animals for short periods of time, which can be a good option if you can't have a long-term pet.

> **THE RESEARCH SAYS . . .**
>
> ### This Is What's Happening in Your Brain and Body
>
> Loneliness is linked to increased inflammatory activity in the body, making you vulnerable to a wide spectrum of health conditions.[8] Your genetics may play a role in your experiences of loneliness, with the heritability rate being roughly 50 percent.[9]
>
> Relational aspects of human interaction such as touch, eye contact, and mirroring have a connection to higher oxytocin levels, a natural "feel good" hormone.[10]

Barriers to Feeling Better

REMOTE WORK

Remote work has become more widely practiced since the COVID-19 pandemic and has many benefits. However, you may find that your interactions with coworkers have lessened, and are largely taking place in online chats, emails, or video calls. You are not alone in this; employee loneliness is at an all-time high.[7]

SOCIAL ANXIETY

Fear that you will be negatively judged during social interactions can lead to feeling lonely. You may be hesitant to initiate or follow up with social interactions, and as a result, lose out on developing strong connections.

It's helpful to remember that the anxiety is happening as a means of self-protection and doesn't always indicate an actual threat. You deserve to have safe, fun, and secure connections (see also chapter 4).

SOCIAL MEDIA

It's ironic that social media platforms invented to connect us to others often have the opposite impact. Social media use increases feelings of loneliness,[11] although research also demonstrates that when used intentionally, it can actually decrease loneliness.[12]

Social media use that increases feelings of loneliness often relates to intensity (seeking out and using social media as a primary support), rumination (having difficulty detaching from what you see on social media), and social comparison.[13]

Using social media to decrease your loneliness takes deliberate effort, but it is possible. Try curating the list of who you follow to be people you truly want to connect with (social pruning),[14] limiting the amount of time you spend on it,[15] and sharing your thoughts and feelings honestly instead of your "highlights reel."[16]

HEALTH ISSUES

Health issues may restrict your ability to go out and be social or may lead you to cancel or put off scheduling plans with friends. If this describes you, chapter 20 may be a good resource. Some communities offer groups and other connection resources if you are experiencing chronic pain or other specific diagnoses.

LACK OF FINANCES

Socialization is often centered around activities that cost money, and if you don't have the financial resources available to take part, you may find yourself withdrawing and feeling lonely.

Sharing your financial concern with others can often help tremendously. While it can feel vulnerable to share that you can't afford to spend money, you may find your friends have been thinking the same thing.

Going for a walk or hike, spending time at the local library, attending free museum days, volunteering at an animal shelter, and joining or forming a book club are some examples of free social activities you might try.

MAKING FRIENDS AS AN ADULT CAN BE HARD

As an adult, you don't always have easy access to a large, diverse peer group like you did when you were in school. Your coworkers may be potential friend options, although if you're looking for connections outside of work, more effort may be needed.

If you're still scratching your head to figure out what could be getting in the way of quality relationships, check out chapter 10 to see what resonates with you.

> **THE RESEARCH SAYS . . .**
>
> ### You May Also Experience These Things
>
> Loneliness has been associated with higher rates of clinically significant depression (page 8), anxiety (page 19), and suicidal ideation.[17] If you live with intense social anxiety and overuse social media, you may experience greater levels of loneliness.[18]
>
> Experiencing deficits in your social needs has been associated with a 29 percent increased risk of coronary heart disease and 32 percent increased risk of stroke.[19]

How to Communicate About Loneliness

IF YOU'RE THE ONE EXPERIENCING LONELINESS

Reach out to your supports regularly. Schedule phone or video chats. Even if you feel like you have nothing to share, you can be present and listen! You can also share that you are grateful for their presence in your life.

Consider what feels like a meaningful social interaction to you and ask if your loved one can provide that. Is it putting all electronics away for a bit? If yes, try saying, "I'm working on being present and I would love for you to join me. Let's put away our phones and be together."

IF A LOVED ONE IS EXPERIENCING LONELINESS

Check on them! Ask them what would feel like meaningful time together and make it happen, within reason. Consider asking them, "Are there any hobbies that you'd like to do? We can check to see what's available in your neighborhood," or "How would you like for me to support you in building more friendships in the area?" Don't just assume your loved one is lonely because they like to spend time alone. Everyone's personality is different, and some people need more time on their own than others. Being alone can be healthy; feeling alone is not.

IF THE PERSON EXPERIENCING LONELINESS IS A CHILD

Children are dependent on the adults around them, and the skills they learn in childhood are likely to stay with them well into adulthood. This could be an opportunity for you and your child to build connections together! Can you schedule a playdate for your child that allows you and the other parent to connect, too? Make sure to listen to your child's desires in this. Children shouldn't be forced to connect with people they don't want to any more than adults should.

What Coping with Loneliness Can Look Like in Real Life

Julian moved to another city right as the COVID-19 pandemic hit and he didn't get an opportunity to connect with anyone in his area. Lockdown was much longer than anyone originally predicted, and even as the quarantine lifted and the world went back to some kind of normal, he wasn't able to establish new connections.

It's been hard for Julian to move out of the routine of being at home and not interacting with others in person. He's also been working from home since then, and only interacting with his coworkers virtually. It's not the meaningful social connection he's craving.

Remote work has been convenient, although Julian's noticed that days will go by before he realizes that he hasn't been outside. Most of his shopping is done online, so it's made going to the store irrelevant. His most meaningful interaction is with the person who delivers his packages.

He talks to his longtime friends occasionally, although it's been harder to make those calls. Everyone is busy, and he feels like he has nothing to share. He starts to realize that he feels lonely.

Julian thinks, *Maybe I should talk to someone about this*. He reaches out to a therapist and starts meeting with them virtually. He talks about not having meaningful social connections, and he realizes that he's been experiencing depression.

As part of his healing, Julian moves the virtual sessions to a hybrid of virtual and in person. He wants to get more comfortable interacting with others in person again, as he realizes that he's been experiencing some anxiety about that, too. Therapy is a safe space to build those skills again and feel more confident. In time, he reaches out to his longtime friends to strengthen those relationships. He finds that they are excited to hear from him. He vows to make an effort to go see them.

With the help of his therapist, Julian also identifies a neighborhood organization in which he gets a weekly opportunity to hang out with his neighbors. Slowly, but surely, he begins to feel like himself again. He is building a good support system in his area and connecting deeper to the support he already has.

READING LIST AND OTHER RESOURCES

Let's Talk About Loneliness: The Search for Connection in a Lonely World by Simone Heng is a helpful guide to understanding the impact of loneliness in the modern age, and what to do about it.

Seek You: A Journey Through American Loneliness by Kristen Radtke is a graphic novel exploring the theme of loneliness, including the history and science behind it.

The Stranger in the Woods by Michael Finkel is a true story about a man who lived as a hermit for twenty-seven years. This book explores both the challenges of being alone and the benefits that can come from spending time alone intentionally.

National Alliance of Mental Illness (nami.org) is a great resource for free groups and meetings on a variety of mental health topics, coping skills, and more.

VolunteerMatch (volunteermatch.org) is an organization that helps connect you with causes in your neighborhood that you care about. It can be a great resource not only to connect with others in your community, but to also put energy towards a cause that is dear to you.

MeetUp (meetup.com) is a social platform that connects you to hobbies or activities you are interested in.

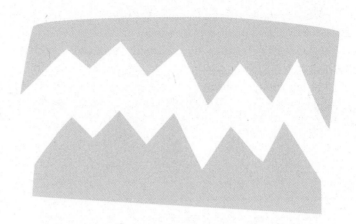

12

WORK STRESS
AND BURNOUT

You likely spend more hours at work than anywhere else, and potentially spend more time with your coworkers than your family and friends. In fact, you may find your manager at work has just as much of an impact on your mental health as your partner, and more than your clinician or therapist.[1] Therefore, it's important to have a safe and supportive work environment.

Being in an unsupportive work environment, receiving poor compensation, or having unrealistic work demands placed on you can cause you strain. Work stress refers to the emotional, physical, or mental negative impact you experience when faced with job demands or expectations, and not having the appropriate resources, support, or knowledge to manage them effectively.[2] With this, you may have trouble concentrating and feel increased self-doubt, irritability, and anxiety. Physically, you may experience headaches, stomach distress, excessive tiredness, or changes in your appetite or weight. You may also procrastinate on work tasks, isolate from loved ones, cancel plans, constantly monitor work emails, see an increase in drinking alcohol or smoking, or experience sleep disruptions.

Burnout is believed to be a result of chronic workplace stress that has not been successfully managed. With burnout, you may experience feelings of energy depletion or exhaustion, feel increased mental distance from your job or have feelings of negativism or cynicism related to it, and a sense of ineffectiveness and lack of accomplishment.[3] Burnout can negatively impact your quality of life.

> **THE RESEARCH SAYS . . .**
>
> ## You Are Not Alone
>
> In the US, 120,000 deaths each year have been reported to be caused by work stress.[4] More than 80 percent of US workers report experiencing work-related stress, with more than 50 percent of those reporting that it has negatively impacted their home life.[5] In a 2023 study spanning ten countries, 60 percent of people said work stress was the biggest factor impacting their mental health.[6]

Strategies to Try

SET BOUNDARIES AT WORK

Having clear start and end times for work can be important in creating a healthy work-life balance. This may be challenging in certain work environments, but it's nevertheless important to prioritize your health and well-being.

If you work from home, create a designated workspace to whatever extent you can. Even if it's just a small desk and a chair in the corner, make that space only for work. Tossing a sheet over the desk or adding a room divider can create more separation.

If possible, take your work email off your personal phone. If you can't, consider turning off notifications entirely, or during your off-hours.

ESTABLISH A ROUTINE

Creating structure can help you manage your to-dos and establish healthy habits. Consider scheduling breaks into your calendar, particularly if you find that you struggle with self-care (like eating lunch) during your workday.

If you work from home, have a similar morning routine as though you were going into the office. Wash your face, change your clothes, and get your work mug ready for the day. Also, create an end-of-day routine, such as taking a walk to create some distance so you can enter your home again with a refreshed mindset.

CLARIFY YOUR JOB'S EXPECTATIONS

Having a clear understanding of how your supervisors are measuring your performance against the duties of your position is helpful. If it's unclear, request a copy of your job description and expectations, and if you have a quarterly or yearly review of your work performance, take that opportunity to discuss your job role expectations.

If there are no expectations, create some yourself based on what you do already and then write a description of reasonable duties and expectations for your position. Talk with your manager or HR department (if there is one) about this.

TAKE ADVANTAGE OF AN EMPLOYEE ASSISTANCE PROGRAM

Some companies offer an Employee Assistance Program (EAP), which provides you with a certain number of free therapy sessions. You can continue meeting with the EAP therapist after your allotted number of sessions have been met; although check to see if they accept your standard insurance plan, or what their self-pay rate is.

DON'T FORGET TO TAKE GOOD CARE OF YOURSELF

When you're feeling overworked, it's easy to not engage in your usual self-care routines. Be mindful to continue eating well, going to bed at a reasonable hour to ensure you get sufficient sleep, make time to exercise, connect with friends, and engage in your hobbies.

CONSIDER CHANGING JOBS

Finding a new job is no small thing. However, if you've tried several boundary-setting strategies and there's no relief, your work environment may be causing too much emotional, physical, and mental damage—and chances are that the company's culture won't be fixed any time soon. In this case, the solution may be to leave your job.

This can be scary, as it involves the unknown. Hopefully, what you do know is that your health and well-being are of the utmost importance.

If you have the flexibility, you may decide to take a job that pays less or is less prestigious in order to have a better quality of life. This is a personal decision, although one with which more people are becoming comfortable. Worldwide, 81 percent of people say they would choose to prioritize their mental health over income, with 64 percent being willing to take a pay cut to work in a job that supports their mental health.[7]

We understand that being able to leave a position is often a luxury. If you can't foresee this in the near future, we hope you know that you are worth doing so if the opportunity arises.

Barriers to a Healthy Work-Life Balance

TOXIC ACHIEVEMENT CULTURE

Having unreasonable expectations placed on you, whether by managers or yourself, can negatively impact all aspects of your life. Prioritizing achievements over your health and well-being reinforces negative beliefs that you are not enough, that it's not safe to say what you need, and leads you to not care for yourself in the necessary ways. On a daily basis, make efforts to identify reasons you are enough that are not related to external achievements.

LACK OF SUPPORT

With unreasonable expectations often comes lack of support, which can lead you to feeling isolated and unable to ask for what you need.

Set your own internal parameters for what constitutes success at work and identify downtimes when you will prioritize rest. Even with external unreasonable expectations, having a clear picture of what is realistically achievable and holding yourself to that can help minimize the feeling that you aren't doing enough.

American society is built on capitalism, which typically values productivity and outcomes over individual needs. Therefore, it's important to honor your limits and boundaries. You deserve rest, self-care, and fun because you're not a machine; you're a person deserving of good things. Identify downtimes during which you will prioritize rest.

A HIGH-STRESS WORK ENVIRONMENT

Working in environments that are unpredictable or involve life-or-death situations can make it challenging to find internal or external peace at work, and even at home. It may be helpful to discuss ways of supporting each other with your colleagues, or to have practices in place to represent the barrier between your personal and work life at the end of each day. For example, try washing your hands before you leave work and imagine yourself "washing off the day," and then change clothes as soon as you get home to further represent the separation between work and home life. Having a "buffer" time during which you exercise, talk to a loved one on the phone, or work on a creative outlet before settling into your evening can also help you transition between work and home.

VICARIOUS TRAUMA

Vicarious trauma is the emotional and mental impact you may experience if you are exposed to trauma at work. You are more likely to experience this if you work in a profession where you regularly witness trauma happening to others, such as medicine, emergency services, mental health, child welfare, law enforcement, or criminal justice.

Feeling as though you're helpless in the face of trauma happening to someone else makes you more vulnerable to vicarious trauma. Feeling empowered to help that person, however, protects you from it. Identify ways in which you can work to reduce the causes of the vicarious trauma. An example could be raising awareness of crisis support lines in your community to help those experiencing a mental health crisis. At work, clearly defining your role in your own mind can help you focus on the ways in which you can help, instead of the ways in which you cannot. Just like some professionals wear protective gear to work, consider the emotional protective "gear" you need to put on each day, including clear boundaries, support from your supervisor, and even therapy if needed, to protect yourself from vicarious trauma at work.

COMPASSION FATIGUE

Compassion fatigue describes the lowered bandwidth you feel for providing care, empathy, and compassion to others after continuous experiences of being present to others' trauma and pain without effective ways to help them. It may be helpful for those providing care to seek care of their own, such as talk therapy, and to set internal boundaries, such as telling yourself it's okay not to over-empathize with those you care for. Understanding the difference between empathy (feeling the person's pain) and compassion (feeling *for* someone from a boundaried distance), and operating from a place of compassion instead of empathy when possible, can be key to preventing compassion fatigue.

IMPOSTER SYNDROME

Imposter syndrome (or imposter phenomenon) is linked to burnout, particularly among the helping professions.[8] It causes you to question your intelligence and abilities, be unable to fully recognize your accomplishments, and overall feel like a fraud.[9] This wear and tear on your self-worth and self-perception can weaken your mental and emotional resources. Make efforts to routinely identify evidence supporting your competence and be mindful not to let negative thinking lead you to discount your qualifications.

WORK-RELATED TRAVEL

You may thrive in the hustle and bustle of work travel, or you may find yourself feeling drained from not sleeping in your own bed, constantly eating out, and always being on the go. If possible, be strategic about how much travel you agree to do and try to schedule the travel so that you have time to recuperate at home between trips.

LONG HOURS, A CONSTANTLY CHANGING SCHEDULE, OR NIGHT WORK

Having an inconsistent work schedule, such as going from day to night shifts, can make it challenging for your body to acclimate as your sleep schedule is disturbed. The winter months can be more challenging if you are impacted by Seasonal Affective Disorder. You may experience increased anxiety, lowered mood, and disconnection from loved ones. Overall, an inconsistent work schedule doesn't provide consistency in getting your needs met. Try to establish routines within the inconsistency. If your shifts frequently change, make efforts to check in with loved ones at some point in your day, to eat healthy meals, and to find time to focus on self-care.

REMOTE WORK

While you may have more flexibility working from home, you also have the disadvantage of not receiving the level of in-person support that you need, and you may experience a blurring of your work and personal life. Keep these areas of life as separate as you can, both in your physical space, if possible, and with your time-related boundaries. Have regular check-ins with your colleagues, friends, and family to reduce feelings of isolation.

How to Communicate About Work Stress or Burnout

IF YOU'RE THE ONE EXPERIENCING WORK STRESS OR BURNOUT

Be open and honest about the boundaries and support you need. You may say something like, "I am working to take back some more of my time. If I am canceling plans with you or spending time checking emails and messages when we're together, please gently point it out. I am working on respecting my time, and yours."

At work, this may be, "I am available during the hours of 9 AM to 5 PM during the workweek and will not be responding to emails or phone calls before or after those hours. These are my hours according to my job description and contract."

When you set a boundary but don't keep it, you are breaking a promise to the most important person: you.

IF A LOVED ONE IS EXPERIENCING WORK STRESS OR BURNOUT

Check in with your loved one and gently (but strongly) encourage them to prioritize their health. Consider using the following questions and prompts.

- How can I support you right now?

- If I was the one experiencing what you're experiencing, what would you tell me? How would you support me? Why are you less important than me?

- Let's schedule some days off and plan to do a relaxing activity together.

What Burnout Can Look Like in Real Life

Ashton has worked five years at their job and has taken two vacations during that time. They work even when they're sick, and those days when they really can't work, they feel guilt and anxiety over what work they're missing. Since their company hasn't added any more of the desperately needed employees to lessen the workload, even after several requests for more support, they are unable to ask a coworker for backup.

Ashton was drawn to this job because the managers talked about how they prioritize a healthy work-life balance and are open to feedback. Although over time, Ashton's realized that the true priority is their daily work output and their managers' unspoken expectation is for them to be immediately available, even after 5 PM.

There is no true support or work-life balance. The long hours, constant need to check their phone and always be available, and relentless work demands have disrupted Ashton's sleep, lowered their mood, and led them to feel disconnected. They're experiencing near constant headaches, they feel exhausted all the time, and they've noticed that they've been getting sick a lot more. It's like their body is trying to tell them something that they haven't been able to truly recognize and accept yet.

Eventually, Ashton goes to their primary care clinician to get a physical to see if there's a medical reason for their headaches. It doesn't make sense to be this sick all the time. They're in their thirties and have always been relatively healthy. Their clinician runs some tests and asks them questions about work and life. When the clinician hears about the unreasonable work demands and lack of resources to rest and restore, they discuss with Ashton that it's their medical opinion that they are experiencing burnout, and if changes aren't made, they may end up experiencing serious long-term health issues.

Ashton is prescribed vitamins and given sleep strategies to help restore their physical health. They are also referred to a mental health clinician to help them navigate these stressors, create boundaries, and uncover what type of work environment they need for their optimal health. It's during this appointment that they realize that their physical, mental, and emotional health are most important, and they are ready to put themself first.

READING LIST AND OTHER RESOURCES

Burnout: The Secret to Unlocking the Stress Cycle by Emily Nagoski and Amelia Nagoski is an amazing book on how you may experience burnout and provides tangible steps you can take to manage stress and return to yourself.

Reducing Secondary Traumatic Stress: Skills for Maintaining a Career in the Helping Professions by Brian Miller is an excellent guide with practical strategies for caring for vicarious trauma, compassion fatigue, and burnout.

The Worklife Coach Podcast features episodes about burnout, imposter phenomenon, and creating a work life that is actually fulfilling.

The *Work Life* podcast by organizational psychologist Adam Grant includes interviews with professionals about numerous work-related topics.

The Secret Thoughts of Successful Women: Why Capable People Suffer from the Imposter Syndrome and How to Thrive in Spite of It by Valerie Young breaks down five different roles that are often found in women who experience imposter syndrome.

Young also discusses imposter phenomenon on the *Ten Percent Happier* podcast, episode 574, "Do You Feel Like an Imposter?"

Soul is an animated film that's not just for kids! It has multiple messages, such as life has meaning beyond work and that we are inherently enough.

For more resources, see page 215.

13

GRIEF

G rief is an inescapable, universal experience, and is often described as the longing for something or someone that we have lost. From losing a sense of safety to losing a loved one, the feeling of grief can be profound and affect you on a mental, emotional, and physical level.[1] Grief isn't limited to after the loss of a loved one or the end of a relationship, it can occur in anticipation of a loss (anticipatory grief).

It's common for past grief to surface when you're experiencing "new" grief, as well as during celebratory occasions, like holidays or life milestones. You may also experience grief related to many topics written about in this book. With depression, you may grieve the loss of time or your sense of self. In trauma, a loss of safety and trust can occur, and you may grieve a previously felt sense of safety and ease in trusting others.

Mary-Francis O'Connor, author of *The Grieving Brain*, talks about grief as a process of learning; learning new ways to navigate your day, new routines, and new ways of being.[2] Grief may be an avenue to build a new sense of self, discovering new meaning in life, or getting in touch with what is truly important. Healing doesn't mean you'll say, "Grief doesn't bother me anymore!" More likely, it will be, "I see you, grief, and we can coexist."

What Professional Treatment May Look Like

Many people find that they don't need professional grief treatment; they simply need time and space to be with their grief. However, there may be a point when grief impacts you so deeply and for a significant period of time that it becomes a mental health concern. In this case, you may be experiencing Prolonged Grief Disorder (PGD),[3] also known as complicated grief. For PGD in adults, the loss occurred at least a year ago, and for children, at least six months. Symptoms occur within the past month and may include deep loneliness, challenges in reengaging in life (connecting with friends or thinking and planning for the future), feeling numb, a sense that life has no meaning, avoidance of reminders of the loss, and intense feelings of anger, bitterness, or sadness.

If you are looking for professional support, you have a variety of options. If you enjoy body work, Sensorimotor Therapy (page 21) may be appealing. Art therapy may be an avenue to express your grief creatively. Cognitive Behavior Therapy can help both adults and children navigate their grief-related thoughts and feelings, particularly if anxiety or depression is also present.[4] Treatment for complicated or enduring grief involves processing the pain of your loss while also reaching acceptance and finding meaning and purpose in life as it is now.[5]

Strategies to Try

LEARN TO RIDE THE WAVES

Grief comes and goes like waves. Some days, the waves are gentle, on others, they are giant and knock you off your feet. An awareness of the unpredictability of grief is an important part of healing. On those gentle days, let yourself laugh and remember the goodness of life. On the tsunami days, it's fine to curl up under the covers and cry. The wisdom of riding the waves is that the pain will ease, and you'll enjoy life again.

JOURNAL

Journaling is a means of processing loss at your own pace by taking time to reflect and to put words to your experiences.

Journaling prompts that you may find helpful include the following.

- How did I learn to process grief in my family?

- What's been modeled to me?

- Has the loss changed what I find to be important?

- Am I avoiding talking about the loss?

- In what ways have I changed since the loss?

- Am I allowing others to support me?

- What would I like my "new normal" to be following this grief?

THE RESEARCH SAYS . . .

This Is What's Happening in Your Brain and Body

The mind-body connection is alive and strong during times of grief. Grief can lead to disruptions in your sleep and memory.[7] As we process our emotions, it is important that we remember to eat, sleep, and engage in our social relationships, in an effort to maintain our health.

ATTEND A SUPPORT GROUP

Whether you experienced a death, the end of a relationship, or a loss of physical functioning, talking with others who've experienced similar situations can be therapeutic, as they may have a more intimate understanding of your feelings.

For some, connecting with faith-based practices helps them connect with their loved ones. Others may find solace in spiritual practices.

YOGA AND BREATHWORK

If you are moving nonstop to avoid feeling your grief, slowing down with mindful breathing can be a gentle way of connecting with your body, thoughts, and feelings again. If you've been more sedentary in your grief, movement may be a means of moving the grief through your body. Yoga and mindful breathwork may be helpful in alleviating experiences of grief, improving mood, and bringing you into a space of connectedness.[6]

ENGAGE IN GRIEF RITUALS

Grief rituals allow for sadness and happiness to coexist. You may write a letter to the individual or situation that you've lost, revisit a special location, or keep mementos as a reminder of that connection. You may engage in extra self-care around events like anniversaries, holidays, and birthdays, and find avenues to allow for some of the sadness or anger to release.

In addition, if the relationship with the individual who passed was unhealthy or toxic, you may feel sadness or relief that they are gone and intense anger regarding their treatment of you. One practice that can help is writing a "genuine obituary." Many survivors of child abuse with whom we have worked say that it feels unfair that others will never know those individuals' true natures. Hearing others celebrate a person who hurt you can be painful. Consider writing something that expresses how you truly feel. Afterward, you can burn or bury the writing.

Barriers to Healing from Grief

NOT HAVING ENOUGH TIME TO PROCESS YOUR GRIEF

Taking time to process grief may be more of a luxury than a given. Paid bereavement time from work, if available, is often limited, and may not afford you the time you truly need. It's challenging to process a loss while also juggling all your other responsibilities.

The process of grieving "is not a one-dimensional experience" and the timetable it occurs in is uniquely your own.[8] Grieve as long as you need; it may be for a pocket of time or take place over a number of years.

FEELING LIKE YOU SHOULD "JUST GET OVER IT"

The feeling of just wanting to get through and be done with it is common, whether it comes from you or others. Grief isn't a chore and pushing it down or away only delays healing. If you keep on tucking it under the rug, how long will it be until you trip over it?

SOCIAL AND CULTURAL DYNAMICS

How is grief processed within your family, culture, or religion? Does it align with what you need? These dynamics may impact how you process and feel supported in your grief. Is it possible for you to ask for what you need, even if doing so would be radical in the system in which you live?

ANTICIPATORY GRIEF

When there's an expected loss, such as in the case of a terminal illness like cancer or Alzheimer's disease, you may have a multitude of mixed emotions that can be hard to reconcile. Grieving often begins while your loved one is still alive. After the loss, you may feel profound sadness and relief that your loved one's suffering has ended, although guilt may follow. You may feel relieved that you no longer experience the "Will it be today?" questions.

How to Communicate About Grief

IF YOU'RE THE ONE EXPERIENCING GRIEF

As much as you can, let people know what you need from them, as well as what doesn't help. You might say, "Please don't ask if I'm okay. I just need silence right now. I know you're here for me. I'll talk when I am ready." Or "Distract me. I need a break from all of this." Sometimes in grief, you have absolutely no idea what you need or want or don't want to hear—or find that it changes from minute to minute. Our tolerance to typical life stress can also be pretty low. Lean on your support system and be kind to yourself, as each day or moment may present a different need.

IF A LOVED ONE IS EXPERIENCING GRIEF

Checking in on a loved one immediately after a loss is important. Attending their loved one's funeral is a simple way of showing up for them. Reaching out in tangible and specific ways, such as saying, "I'm having dinner delivered to your house tomorrow night," or "I'm running errands today and would like to take any off your plate while I'm at it," may be better received than open statements like "I'm here for whatever you need." Most people who have experienced losing a loved one say that just hearing "I'm so sorry" and being given a hug can mean everything. Don't worry about having a perfect response to your loved one's grief; acknowledging it and not ignoring it is the most important thing.

Continue checking in on a loved one long after a loss. Grieving doesn't necessarily end, it can show up randomly or around anniversaries, holidays, and other special occasions. You may say, "Hey, I know their birthday is coming up and I recognize that it may be a pretty emotional time. I'd love to be there for you in any way that I am able," or "I'm here if you want to talk or laugh."

You may fear that bringing up a loss will be too painful for the person experiencing it. However, they are likely thinking of their loss daily, and knowing someone else remembers and is thinking of it, too, can be a solace. Simply being present with someone can also be meaningful. Your loving presence can speak volumes.

IF THE PERSON EXPERIENCING GRIEF IS A CHILD

Grief is a natural process, but because our culture doesn't always support it, children may need to be told that it's okay to grieve.

Having photos on display of the person or pet you are grieving can help. Consider making a photo book for your child so they can have a memento to help them grieve. The process will likely help you, too.

Modeling is an important part of helping a child develop good mental health. If your child sees you expressing your feelings, they will know that they can do so, too. Parents often think that their children need to see them be strong and not cry, but that's not true. Children need to see you express your feelings in appropriate ways, and also to learn that their difficult feelings won't last forever because they will see that you are okay again after your tears.

While crying or expressing other emotions in front of children is healthy, be mindful that they don't take on responsibility for your feelings. Saying "I feel sad, and it's okay that I feel sad. I know how to take care of myself when I am feeling sad" can help with this balance.

What Grieving Can Look Like in Real Life

Amanda's grandmother spent the last two months of her life in hospice care at Amanda's parents' house. They were initially told that she had days to live, but she held strong for weeks. At times, it didn't seem like she was near the end of her life at all—she seemed vibrant and ate everything in sight. It was as though her family coming together to support her had revitalized her. The family often questioned whether she was near the end or not, and it was easy to forget that she was sick. When reality returned, it felt shocking. Amanda was determined to soak up every moment with her that she could, while also grieving the inevitable loss.

The visible decline happened in the last two weeks of her grandmother's life. During this time, it felt hard to rest as Amanda was constantly on the alert. The "on edge" feeling was taxing, as was witnessing her grandmother needing more care. Amanda's once larger-than-life grandmother was so fragile, and Amanda took care of her in all the ways her grandmother had taken care of her as a child. Amanda and her family were by her side as she passed away and were grateful that she was finally at rest.

It didn't truly hit Amanda until the day of the funeral that her grandmother was gone. She was so focused on being a caregiver and once that was done, there was room for all her feelings. She found that other family members felt the same way, and as a result, she didn't feel alone. Amanda knew that the grieving process often ebbed and flowed, and that it was normal to sometimes feel as though the loss hadn't happened.

The first year of holidays and birthdays were tough, and Amanda found that honoring her grandmother in little ways—like having her grandmother's favorite dessert on her birthday—helped to ease the pain. Looking at pictures and reflecting on the impact of her grandmother on her life also helped. Amanda noticed that the sadness would creep in on some days, and she would take time to acknowledge it. She knew that avoiding her grief wouldn't help her, as hard as it was sometimes to face, and that the grieving wouldn't necessarily have an end point. The reality was that she'd never stop missing her grandmother, and that meant their love would always stay alive, too.

READING LIST AND OTHER RESOURCES

It's OK That You're Not OK: Meeting Grief and Loss in a Culture That Doesn't Understand by Megan Devine gives helpful information about what grief can look like, and permission to grieve in the way you need. If you or a loved one is freshly grieving, this is the book for you.

The Grieving Brain: The Surprising Science of How We Learn from Love and Loss by Mary-Frances O'Connor is a resource for understanding how our brains are impacted both by the development and loss of attachment.

The Grief Practice by Monique Minahan is both a book to guide you through grief and a website (thegriefpractice.com) with many resources, including yoga practices and body scans.

Memoirs about grief such as *The Year of Magical Thinking* by Joan Didion, *The Light of the World* by Elizabeth Alexander, and *In Love: A Memoir of Love and Loss* by Amy Bloom can help you feel connected to others who have experienced grief of many kinds.

Terrible, Thanks for Asking with Nora McInerny, *All There Is* with Anderson Cooper, *Breathing Wind* with Naila Francis and Sarah Davis, and *Everything Happens* with Kate Bowler are all podcasts in which the hosts invite you to journey with them as they explore their own experiences with loss of all kinds and interview others who have experienced grief as well.

Grief Share (griefshare.org) is a church-based nondenominational grief group that meets all over the country.

The Endless Story: Explaining Life and Death to Children by Melissa Kircher is a beautiful book that invites children to explore grief and traditions around grieving.

Inside Out is an animated film about one girl's journey grieving and accepting a loss after moving from the home she's always known and having to start over. It also highlights various emotional experiences in a child-accessible way, and the messages hit home for adults as well!

I Miss You: A First Look at Death by Pat Thomas is a children's book that provides age-appropriate language for talking about loss with a child as well as questions to help children explore their feelings.

3

SEXUAL HEALTH

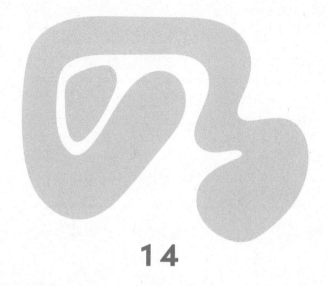

14

INFERTILITY AND PREGNANCY LOSS

ssues related to infertility and pregnancy loss are often borne silently by those who experience them. Both infertility and miscarriage affect many people and yet are rarely talked about or acknowledged in our society. If you have experienced infertility or pregnancy loss, you may be grieving, and you may feel alone. Your experiences may be taking a toll on your relationships. You may find yourself feeling anxious, depressed, or even hopeless about the future. You may feel angry that your reproductive journey was not what you expected, or what your friends or family experienced. You are allowed to feel angry and instead of repressing or avoiding your anger, try inviting it to speak to you by journaling, scribbling, or even screaming. Think of anger as a storm passing by.

Living in the twenty-first century, we think of ourselves as enlightened about reproductive health. You likely know the choices available to you, choices that range from delaying childbearing or choosing to build a family through medical or social options. While abortion rights remain hotly contested in the US, at the time of the publication of this book, studies suggest that abortion numbers actually rose since the reversal of *Roe v. Wade*, part of an ever-changing landscape of reproductive rights.[1] You can have successful pregnancies after transitioning your gender, you can create families by numerous means other than giving birth, and childbirth and child rearing are choices that you can make rather than foregone conclusions. "Childfree" people have chosen to remain childless for various reasons.

Despite all of this progress, the fact remains that numerous issues may impact you when trying to have a successful pregnancy, and that a fertility journey can have a significant impact on your mental health.

> ## THE RESEARCH SAYS . . .
>
> ### You Are Not Alone
>
> It's estimated that one in five persons with a uterus in the United States experience infertility, meaning they've been unable to conceive after one year of trying.[2] As many as 25 percent of pregnancies in developed countries end in miscarriage.[3]
>
> In heterosexual couples trying to conceive, as much as 50 percent of infertility is connected to the male partner.[4] Despite this fact, much of the research focusing on the impact of infertility on mental health analyzes women without considering men. Perhaps not surprisingly then, men report feeling isolated and "emasculated" by their experience of infertility.[5]

What Professional Treatment Can Look Like

While we cannot help you with your medical fertility journey, the rest of this chapter is meant to help support your mental health as you process pregnancy loss or infertility. If you need help communicating with a medical professional, please turn to chapter 25.

COGNITIVE BEHAVIORAL THERAPY

Because infertility often results in unhelpful thinking, such as *There is something wrong with me*, or *I will never get to have the family I want*, Cognitive

Behavioral Therapy can be an effective treatment for coping with the mental health impact of infertility.[6]

EYE MOVEMENT DESENSITIZATION AND REPROCESSING

Both infertility and miscarriage have been linked to causing Post-Traumatic Stress Disorder, and the symptoms associated with reproductive trauma have been found to be reduced with Eye Movement Desensitization and Reprocessing (EMDR).[7]

Strategies to Try

COMMEMORATE YOUR LOSS

When people die, we have rituals, like funerals, that help us acknowledge our grief. All too often, pregnancy-related losses are not commemorated. Whether you need to process the pain of never being able to conceive, the painful journey it took to conceive, or the anguish of losing a pregnancy, consider doing something that will commemorate your experience.

This can include holding a small memorial alone or with loved ones. You could bury something that was precious to you on the journey, such as a pregnancy test or baby item. You may choose to read a poem, or to journal about the life you had hoped for with a baby. Or perhaps you could get a tattoo or buy yourself a piece of jewelry or art that expresses how meaningful this loss was to you. Whatever you choose, honoring what you went through can be part of healing.

GIVE YOURSELF TIME

It can be hard to give yourself permission to be fully with your grief. However, doing so is an important part of healing and helps to prevent developing the complicated grief that can arise when we don't allow the natural process to take place.

You may find it hard to grieve, especially if it's been some time since your loss. Sometimes music helps us connect with our grief. A song such as "Bigger Than the Whole Sky" by Taylor Swift, can give you a sense that you are not alone in your grief. You may want to listen to music that you know helps you connect with grief, and then invite yourself to express your feelings through tears, which are our body's natural way of releasing emotion (for more, see chapter 13).

ENGAGE IN MIND-BODY PRACTICES

If you're experiencing infertility, there may be some benefit to your overall mental health in practicing mind-body interventions such as mindfulness and yoga.[8] It's important not to use such practices as checklist items, strategies you think may help result in a successful pregnancy, or as another way to measure your worth. Instead, use these methods as tools for self-understanding, as a way to get in touch with your body and what it may need or want independent of pregnancy.

See what happens when you try connecting with yourself on the yoga mat to simply notice your body, breathe into it mindfully, and offer it what it needs, whether that's gentle movement, loving touch, or words of affirmation.

TALK ABOUT IT

Whether you go to therapy, find a support group, join an online community, or have a good friend who listens and understands, don't sit alone with this heartache. Give yourself permission to process out loud what these experiences have been like, and for your pain to be witnessed.

Things That Can Make Coping with Infertility or Pregnancy Loss Harder

SOCIAL PRESSURE AND STIGMA

Despite how far we may have come in understanding childbearing as a choice, you may still feel pressure from family members or your social circles to have children, or stigma related to not having children.[9] Subconscious messaging about how having children is linked to your self-worth and life's success can further complicate the already complex fertility journey as you decide what choices are best for you.

You may decide you need to set boundaries around what pregnancy-related topics are and are not okay for people to talk to you about. (For more about setting boundaries, see page 104.)

FEELINGS OF SOCIAL ISOLATION

Men can experience both the medical and emotional impact of infertility and miscarriage. Because men's role in infertility is discussed less, if you are a male experiencing infertility, you may have an increased sense of isolation or inferiority in relation to your peers.[10] And due to the silence that often surrounds reproductive health, you may struggle to reach out for support regardless of your gender identity.

MEDICAL RACISM AND INSTITUTIONAL EXCLUSION

In general, white, cisgender women and heterosexual couples have been centered in the research and treatment of reproductive concerns, to the detriment of other races, genders, and identities.[11] Marginalized communities experience disproportionate obstacles and trauma during their reproductive health journeys. Black people are often the victims of medical racism, which has led to tragic outcomes in pregnancy and childbirth.[12] The lack of research in addition to the reproductive world's institutional exclusion of the LGBTQ+ community creates numerous barriers for those weighing up their reproductive options, including through discrimination and lack of informed health care.[13] Reproductive justice is a movement that seeks to center the experiences and needs of marginalized communities in order to create equitable reproductive health care access and options.

INSENSITIVE TREATMENT

The way the medical community discusses and treats infertility and miscarriage can be problematic. Many clients have told us they felt shocked when they read the words "spontaneous abortion" on their medical paperwork following a miscarriage. While the medical community refers to a miscarriage as a spontaneous abortion, the association between abortion and choice can make that terminology upsetting if you have experienced a loss you would have done anything to prevent.

Additionally, medical professionals may have treated your infertility or miscarriage only as a medical problem, not as an experience that can cause grief or trauma. While it is not the role of most medical

THE RESEARCH SAYS . . .

You May Also Experience These Things

Women experiencing infertility are significantly more likely to experience depression (page 8) than women in the general population, and women who have had recurrent miscarriages experience much more anxiety (page 19) than women with low miscarriage risk.[14] Cortisol levels, which indicate stress, are higher in women undergoing in-vitro fertilization than in the general female population.[15]

professionals to comment on the mental health impact of a medical issue, the absence of consideration, along with the absence of understanding or empathy from loved ones, can make you feel alone and misunderstood.

The medical procedures you may go through when you're experiencing infertility or miscarriage can cause pain and even trauma. Whether you have to get constant blood work as part of your fertility treatment, or a D&C (dilation and curettage) after a miscarriage, it's likely you've experienced these procedures in cold, clinical settings while internally you were suffering.

To bring yourself some comfort in these settings, consider bringing a loved one with you if you can, making a playlist of soothing music to listen to the whole time, wearing the coziest clothing you own, or treating yourself to comfort food to help your body feel a little more nourished.

How to Communicate About Infertility and Pregnancy Loss

IF YOU'RE THE ONE EXPERIENCING LOSS RELATED TO PREGNANCY

Don't be afraid to share how this loss feels with your loved ones. While it may not be fair to bear the responsibility of expressing your grief to others, the reality is that emotional pain related to infertility and pregnancy loss is so misunderstood that you may need to share your experiences to get support. If it feels too hard to say aloud, see if you can text your feelings. If you can't put how you feel into words, try sharing this chapter with them.

IF A LOVED ONE IS EXPERIENCING LOSS RELATED TO PREGNANCY

Don't tell the person experiencing infertility or miscarriage that it was "meant to be." Statements that minimize the emotional and social pain of the experience in favor of pointing out that there are medical or social benefits are not helpful. Neither is giving medical advice; people experiencing fertility-related loss have usually tried every medical option available. Instead, try saying things like "I'm so sorry that happened to you. You don't deserve this," or "I can only imagine how hard that is to go through. I'm here to listen."

You might also consider sending a meal or flowers, as you would for other losses. Actions like these communicate to the person experiencing pregnancy-related loss that their experience matters.

And make sure you include all partners in your expressions of support.

What Coping with Infertility and Pregnancy Loss Can Look Like in Real Life

Ryan always planned to have children, and after setting up her other life goals for success, she set her sights on family planning. Months go by, and she finds herself unable to conceive. She's heard how important it is to avoid stress when trying to get pregnant, so she tries her hardest to keep herself calm. However, it seems the harder she tries, the more anxious she feels. Her ob-gyn tells her there is nothing she can do until she's gone a whole year without conceiving. Eventually, she is able to receive an infertility diagnosis and she decides to undergo in-vitro fertilization (IVF).

The IVF process is grueling. Ryan uses up all her savings and her body feels terrible on the medication used to help her produce more eggs for harvesting. Because of the medication's side effects, it's hard to focus at work, and she feels irritable all the time. Every time she has an unsuccessful IVF outcome, Ryan feels herself getting more depressed. Finally, the IVF is successful, and she feels she can breathe.

Ryan buys baby clothes and picks out a crib, but at eleven weeks she loses the pregnancy. She wonders if she did something wrong, or if she just isn't cut out to be a parent. People tell her, "It happened for a reason," that there must have been something wrong with the baby, and every time they do, she wants to scream. It feels like no one understands. She almost doesn't try again, but eventually she tries with the eggs she has left from the last cycle. She has a successful pregnancy this time, and she is so happy and relieved, but even her closest friends don't seem to understand that this doesn't make up for all the pain of the earlier treatments and the baby she lost. Those painful emotions are still with her, even during this happy time.

In an online support group, Ryan finds people who understand what she's been through. Talking about it with others who get how much her body and heart have both suffered helps. She learns to mindfully be with her new baby while also letting herself grieve the one she lost. She learns to speak kindly to her body again after all the time she spent being angry at it for what she blamed it for. She learns to finally treat her body as a friend.

READING LIST AND OTHER RESOURCES

The Retrievals is a podcast that documents the experience of women undergoing IVF at Yale University's fertility clinic. The podcast is a heartbreaking look at the experience of IVF. While the podcast's focus is on a crime that left the women without pain medication for their egg retrievals, the story communicates the desperation and anxiety that often accompany fertility treatment.

World Childless Week (worldchildlessweek.net) is an online resource that hosts webinars, online communities, and other resources if you're experiencing childlessness for a variety of reasons.

Saying Goodbye (sayinggoodbye.org) is an online organization devoted to helping you create remembrance services if you have lost a child during pregnancy, birth, or infancy.

Resolve.org is an organization dedicated to providing support, information, and advocacy if you are going through the process of IVF. They also provide options for community support.

The Childless Collective (childlesscollective.com) provides online support to those struggling with being childless.

We Are Childfree (wearechildfree.com) is a resource dedicated to providing support and encouragement for those who choose to be child-free.

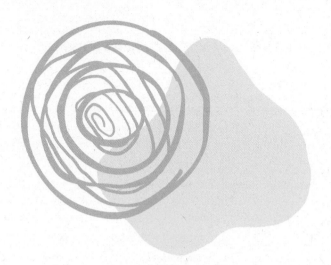

15

SEXUAL
ASSAULT

This chapter discusses many aspects of trauma, in particular sexual trauma. If this causes you distress, be sure to read this chapter in a safe space with healthy self-soothing strategies readily available. If you find that you need to put the book down, please do so. The book will be there for you when you are in a mental and emotional space to read it.

S exual assault is a sexual act committed against someone who does not or cannot consent.[1] According to the Department of Justice, less than 20 percent of sexual assault against adults and less than 10 percent of sexual assault against children is committed by strangers; most people are assaulted by someone they know and trust.[2]

Estimates vary greatly due to differences in and under-reporting, but it's thought that one in every three American women and one in every six American men experiences sexual violence in their lifetime.[3] According to the Rape, Abuse, and Incest National Network (RAINN), every sixty-eight seconds someone in the United States experiences sexual assault.[4]

The prevalence of sexual assault is so extensive that it can be hard to grasp the reality, and yet due to the shame and secrecy that have historically surrounded sexual trauma, many survivors never speak about their experiences. The #MeToo movement that began in 2017 helped many survivors begin to name and speak about their experiences, but the fact remains that sexual assault is shrouded in myths and stigma.

The psychological symptoms in the aftermath of a sexual trauma are numerous and can include hypervigilance (feeling on a constant high alert), dissociation (feeling checked out or emotionally numb), anger, depression, feelings of fear and general unsafety, and self-harm.[5]

What Professional Help May Look Like

If you have experienced a sexual assault at any point in your life, you deserve compassionate trauma-informed care. When you are working with a trauma-informed professional, they should teach you about how your brain and body responded to the trauma. This is an important part of healing. As we like to say, "Psychoeducation is like giving someone the keys to their own car."

A trauma-informed professional can teach you about tonic immobility. Tonic immobility is a powerful survival response during which people (and animals) under extreme stress freeze as if paralyzed. This is an involuntary response and one that scientists view as protective, as the "play dead" response often results in less physical harm.[6] But although the human nervous system means it to be protective, tonic immobility can be cruel to experience, as you remain fully aware of what is happening but unable to do anything about it.

Tonic immobility is twice as likely to occur during child sexual abuse and adult sexual assault than other kinds of trauma.[8] Researchers believe that a tonic immobility response is an important indicator of whether a sexual assault survivor will develop Post-Traumatic Stress Disorder, since it brings with it feelings of shame and guilt.[9] Understanding that tonic immobility is a common nervous system response to sexual assault can help victims and their loved ones find freedom from those feelings.

If you decide you want professional support, here are some options to consider.

EYE MOVEMENT DESENSITIZATION AND REPROCESSING (EMDR) AND TRAUMA-FOCUSED COGNITIVE BEHAVIORAL THERAPY (TF-CBT)

EMDR has been shown to have the most positive impact if you are recovering from sexual assault, with Trauma-Focused Cognitive Behavioral Therapy coming in second.[10] Both are considered frontline treatments for those who have experienced a sexual assault.

DIALECTICAL BEHAVIORAL THERAPY FOR PTSD (DBT-PTSD) AND COGNITIVE PROCESSING THERAPY (CPT)

These are also effective therapies.[11] See the glossary beginning on page 265 for more about these therapies.

Strategies to Try

Determine that you should be receiving trauma-informed treatment and that you can advocate for it if you are not. Being trauma-informed should be approached holistically by well-meaning care clinicians who understand the impact of trauma and the potential for retraumatization.[12] These professionals understand the scientific impact of sexual assault on the brain and body.

UNDERSTAND THAT IT'S NOT LOGICAL, IT'S BIOLOGICAL

If you are a survivor, recognizing how these symptoms are your brain and body's best efforts to protect you is important as you heal. Have you ever heard about how you are supposed to "play dead" if attacked by a grizzly bear? Grizzly bears are "grazers," and if you play dead, they will likely snack on you and then move on, giving you an opportunity to escape, injured but alive. You may wonder how anyone could play dead while being munched on by a grizzly bear, but learning about tonic immobility helps us understand. Living creatures are designed with many defense mechanisms to protect themselves against predators. Some of them are being paralyzed during a sexual assault (the defense mechanism hopes the predator will eventually get tired and leave the victim alone), impairing the ability to recall memory (so that it doesn't have to be relived), and warning you from potential new danger through trauma activation (even when the activators can be totally benign things on their own, like music or a particular color, it's just that they were around at the time of the assault). When you find yourself in these defense mechanisms, remind yourself, "It's not logical, it's biological."

> **THE RESEARCH SAYS . . .**
>
> ### This Is What's Happening in Your Brain and Body
>
> Research has found that sexual assault has numerous physical impacts as well as mental, including but not limited to gastrointestinal disorders and symptoms, reproductive symptoms such as painful intercourse or lack of sexual pleasure, frequent headaches, asthma, neurologic symptoms, sleep disturbances, and chronic pain (see chapters 20 and 21).[13] Much of this is due to the prolonged inflammatory response caused by stress hormones such as cortisol, adrenaline, and norepinephrine, which are released during and in the aftermath of a sexual assault.[14]

ASK FOR ACCOMMODATIONS THAT MAKE YOU FEEL SAFE

Because of all of the medical implications of sexual trauma listed in the "This Is What's Happening in Your Brain and Body" box above, you may find yourself having to attend numerous medical appointments after a sexual assault, from visits directly related to the assault to others years later in the aftermath. It is crucial for sexual assault survivors to have medical care, especially due to poor medical outcomes following trauma as found in the ACE study (page 68). However, many survivors find it difficult to be alone in a room with a medical clinician who is touching them and is perceived to have power over them.

It is always your right to request that another person be present in the room with you during any medical examination or treatment. You can explain that you'd like this to be provided when you schedule your appointment or bring a trusted friend or family member with you.

Some survivors also find it helpful to have a written directive to provide the medical clinician, especially if the care will be complicated, such as surgery, or if it will involve potentially activating things, such as an ID bracelet or IV (feelings of restraint), a hospital gown (feeling unclothed), anesthesia (feelings of paralysis and helplessness), or dental procedures (memories of oral assaults). This can simply be a document you and your therapist or another support person work on together to provide to your medical clinicians prior to treatment. It could include strategies such as having a loose ID bracelet, being permitted to wear loose-fitting street clothes, or being prescribed anti-anxiety medication before a procedure. Give yourself permission to advocate for any strategy that will help you feel safer during your medical procedure and show your clinician this book if you need to help them understand why.

Barriers to Healing from Sexual Assault

DISCOMFORT TALKING ABOUT SEXUAL ASSAULT

Some survivors are uncomfortable with terms such as "rape" and "sexual assault." While there are criminal codes that govern what specific terms mean in the legal system, generally speaking "sexual assault" can refer to a wide variety of sexual trauma. If you're not comfortable with a particular word, it's okay for you to choose a term, such as "sexual trauma" or even just "trauma," that feels more accessible to you.

SOCIETAL MYTHS

Our culture's general lack of awareness about what constitutes sexual assault contributes to the myths, misunderstandings, and general mistreatment of sexual assault survivors. Sexual assault does *not* include only rape or a violent assault by a stranger. In fact, most sexual assault is committed by someone the victim knew and trusted.[15]

CONFUSION AND DENIAL ABOUT THE ASSAULT

Because of the realities of tonic immobility and dissociation, and also the complications of an emotional interpersonal betrayal, many people do not realize they are being assaulted at first, even sometimes long after the assault. This is further complicated for survivors of drug-facilitated sexual assault, in which alcohol or drugs were used to enable the assault, making it difficult for survivors to piece together what happened to them.

A MISUNDERSTANDING OF CONSENT

In a general sense, a sexual assault is when sexual activity of any kind is not consented to by all parties.

To understand true consent, it is important to understand when consent is not present. We used to be taught that "no means no," but because of factors such as tonic immobility, it is now taught that consent must be *informed* (the person fully understands what is being asked of them), *sober* (the decision wasn't made in a state of intoxication from drugs or alcohol), *enthusiastic* (the word "yes" doesn't count if the person's behavior is saying otherwise), and *ongoing* (a person can change their mind at any point and stop).

When we understand consent, we understand that sexual assault can happen in many contexts. Survivors often feel confused when they experience something that felt violating but it has never been included to count as sexual assault. This includes things such as unauthorized pelvic exams in medical settings,[16] "stealthing" (a practice in which a partner removes a condom during intercourse without asking permission),[17] and being coerced into sharing explicit sexual images.

FEAR OF JUDGMENT AND BLAME

You might be hesitant to speak out from fear of facing judgment and blame from others.[18] Well-intentioned friends and family often fall back on old, inaccurate stereotypes when confronted with something as terrible as sexual assault and may question why the victim went out at night, wore certain clothing, or consumed alcohol.

People may ask these questions because they feel helpless when hearing about a loved one being sexually assaulted and are grasping at ways to understand it. Such questions also reflect a desire to be able to place blame, in a misguided (and ineffective) attempt to feel safer themselves.

These kinds of questions lead to more shame and self-blame in survivors who are already trying to cope with what happened. Sexual assault is never the fault of the survivor, and these statements feed into a culture that centers on rapists, telling victims that they need to change their behavior to accommodate them.

How to Communicate About Sexual Assault

IF YOU'RE THE ONE WHO WAS SEXUALLY ASSAULTED
No one should ever have to experience sexual assault. We know how isolating the aftermath can be, and we hope this chapter has made you feel less alone. We also hope that you continue to reach out for the support you need, whether that's therapy, a book, or a support group. If it's within your level of comfort, it may be helpful to speak with a person you trust and to consider telling them what will help you feel supported, such as saying, "Please listen to my story without asking questions."

IF A LOVED ONE WAS SEXUALLY ASSAULTED
Keep in mind that only the survivor can decide what to do with their story, including whether to report it.

Many adult survivors of sexual assault or abuse choose not to report their experience due to fears about the criminal justice process and the mental health impact it may have. Since only 2.5 percent of people who perpetrate sexual assault end up in prison, this is not an unfounded fear.[21]

Other survivors do decide to proceed with reporting their assault, and some find the experience empowering. This choice is deeply personal and depends on a myriad of factors including the support a survivor has for the long and grueling process. It will not be like court cases on TV, and loved ones planning to support someone through a criminal justice process should be prepared for a lengthy process.

You may consider saying to your loved one, "I am so sorry this happened to you. I am here to walk with you through the aftermath, whatever direction you decide to go." Instead of questioning their decisions, consider bringing curiosity to them. For example, "Tell me about what helped you make the decision to report/not report." And it's worth being extra careful about questions or statements that may seem as though you are blaming the victim, who may be feeling sensitive to blame at the moment.

IF THE PERSON WHO WAS SEXUALLY ASSAULTED IS A CHILD

First of all, *believe the child.* Children do not make up being sexually assaulted. Children do not even have the information needed to imagine being sexually assaulted. Too many adult survivors tried telling people when they were children only to be brushed off or disbelieved, resulting in years more of abuse. When a child tells someone of their assault and is not believed, it emboldens the sex offender.

If your child needs to be evaluated, call in the professionals. In most counties in the United States, a trained forensic interviewer at a Child Advocacy Center will interview your child in an age-appropriate way to find out what happened. If you contact your local reporting agency (most states have child abuse reporting hotlines you can call) and your child is going to be interviewed, ask if a Child Advocacy Center is available in your area.

It's never too soon to teach children that their body belongs to them. The "bathing suit rule" is an easy way to introduce the concept, letting young children know that the parts of their bodies covered by a bathing suit are off-limits to anyone except a caregiver who needs to keep them clean or healthy (such as by helping with toileting or giving a medical exam).

However, because abusers will use that language, too, also teach your children that they get to decide what is okay for their bodies, and if anyone, even a family member or clinician, makes them feel uncomfortable, they can say no and tell a different grown-up. Identify multiple grown-ups they can tell. It's important that if you teach your children this, you must enforce it. That means if your child says someone makes them feel uncomfortable, listen and let them have body autonomy. It's impossible to protect every child from sexual abuse but teaching them body autonomy is a good place to start.

If your child has acted out sexually on another child, help is available. Problematic Sexual Behavior (PSB) is on the rise,[22] perhaps due to children's exposure to adult sexual content on TV or online. Children act out what they see, and it is not unusual for young children to act out sexually on other children out of curiosity. Problematic Sexual Behavior-Cognitive Behavioral Therapy is an evidence-based treatment for children displaying PSB.[23] It teaches children the "sexual behavior rules" in age-appropriate ways to learn the rules for respecting other people's bodies, just like they learn the rules to wear a seat belt or cross the street.

What the Aftermath of Sexual Assault Can Look Like in Real Life

Because reading about experiences with sexual assault can be distressing, we've chosen to be general here rather than share a specific case example. Be sure to read this section in a safe space with self-soothing strategies readily available, and feel free to take a break if you need to do so.

Many survivors of sexual trauma report that after the assault it felt like choices were taken out of their hands. Because sexual assault is already a violating experience, continuing this trauma is particularly harmful. If you have been sexually assaulted, reaching out to your local rape crisis center is an important first step, so that you can be connected with resources and advocacy to support you.

Rape crisis center staff are trained to listen nonjudgmentally and to help the survivor decide on the next steps that are best for them. For many, the first recommended step is a medical examination conducted by a trained professional, called a SANE (sexual assault nursing exam) nurse, which ideally will happen within seventy-two hours of the assault. (SANE exams can also be conducted well after seventy-two hours, and you should always reach out to your local rape crisis center for information if you are unsure whether to complete a medical exam.)

While one of the goals of a SANE is to collect forensic evidence in case the survivor decides to move forward with reporting to law enforcement, adults can have a SANE for medical purposes, including STI treatment and to obtain Plan B to prevent pregnancy, without their information being reported to law enforcement.

In the United States, due to mandated reporting laws, professionals who become aware of the sexual assault or abuse of a minor under the age of eighteen must report this information to the authorities in order to protect the child and other potential victims. We also must acknowledge the trauma often caused by the mandated reporting of child abuse. Survivors can be retraumatized by the involvement of the system.

Many sexual assault survivors are surprised by how long the criminal justice process takes; it is not uncommon for a year or two to pass before the case is heard in court. Finding ways to take command of your healing journey despite factors outside of your control may be an important part of recovery.

In many places, including jury trials in the United States, whether or not a victim "fought back" is considered to be important for determining if the assault was consensual or not. Understanding the science of tonic immobility is crucial for survivors trying to heal from their assault, for loved ones trying to understand it, and for the systems trying to determine a legal outcome.[24]

The stress hormones released by the brain during a sexual assault impair memory.[25] Because of this, law enforcement, criminal justice prosecutors, and others need to understand how memory and sexual assault interact in order to have an accurate picture of a survivor's recall and ability to testify. If they do not, it can result in more trauma for the survivor. Utilizing your local rape crisis center will help you find the support and resources you need to get through this process, regardless of the outcome.

> If you or someone you know has been sexually assaulted, reaching out to your local Rape Crisis Center is an important first step. You can find your local center at RAINN.org, or by calling the National Sexual Assault Hotline, 800-656-HOPE.

READING LIST AND OTHER RESOURCES

Know My Name is Chanel Miller's autobiography of her experience being sexually assaulted and the resulting criminal trial. This book helps give a snapshot of what it's like to survive both sexual assault and the US criminal justice system.

Letters to Survivors: Words of Comfort for Women Recovering from Rape edited by Matt Atkinson is a beautifully illustrated book of letters from survivors to survivors. Each letter contains words of wisdom for the healing journey. While, like many resources for survivors of sexual assault, the book is written with women in mind, its words are applicable to those of all genders.

If your sexual trauma is impacting your sexual functioning, *Better Sex Through Mindfulness: How Women Can Cultivate Desire* by Lori Brotto; *Sex Positions For Every Body* by Jill McDevitt; *Healing Painful Sex: A Woman's Guide to Confronting, Diagnosing, and Treating Sexual Pain* by Deborah Coady and Nancy Fish; and *Come as You Are: The Surprising New Science that Will Transform Your Sex Life* by Emily Nagoski are some books to consider in your healing process.

If you identify as a man and have experienced sexual assault, you may find comfort in the organization 1 in 6 (1in6.org), which focuses on bringing awareness to the prevalence of male sexual assault, and to connect male survivors with support.

If you are looking for help for a child who has Problematic Sexual Behavior, you can find more resources at the National Center on the Sexual Behavior of Youth's website (connect.ncsby.org/psbcbt/psbcbt-model/resources).

The Justice Department Office on Violence Against Women (OVW) has a list of local resources and coalitions within each state. See justice.gov/ovw/local-resources.

Tea with a Trauma Therapist (teawithatraumatherapist.com) is an online course developed by Charity O'Reilly (one of this book's authors) to help survivors learn about their trauma responses.

For more resources, see the lists on pages 66 and 76.

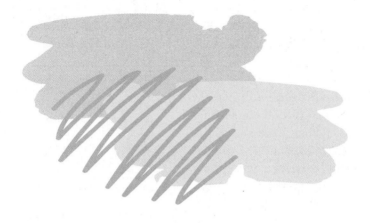

16

INTIMATE PARTNER VIOLENCE

Trust, respect, and safety are foundations of a healthy intimate or romantic relationship. To have the deep sense that you are safe and supported is what allows you to develop a trusting partnership. Unfortunately, this is sometimes lacking within relationships.

Intimate partner violence (IPV) is described as any act—actual or threatened—of physical, sexual, or emotional abuse, as well as controlling and manipulative behaviors within an intimate relationship. These actions can lead to harm on many levels, including physical, sexual, and psychological.[1] Marriage, dating, engagement, and romantic partners are all considered intimate relationships, and you don't need to be living with the abusive individual in order to experience IPV (this is partly why the term "intimate partner violence" is now used instead of "domestic violence").

IPV can take many forms, including physical, sexual, emotional, and financial. Those who engage in IPV likely do so on purpose to gain power and coercive control. You can find the "power and control wheel," which was developed by the Domestic Abuse Intervention Project, online, including on the National Domestic Violence Hotline's website.

Behaviors seen in IPV can range from subtle to overt, although the impact can be the same. You may be left feeling inadequate, unsafe, trapped, confused, traumatized, or as though you have no solid sense of self. It is our hope that if you have experienced or are experiencing IPV, or have a loved one who has, that you feel seen in this chapter and understand that you are not alone, you are not to blame, and that you are supported.

What Professional Help May Look Like

Psychoeducation—learning about what IPV is and how it impacts you—is an important part of professional treatment. You may benefit from learning more about the dynamics of power and control, how trauma impacts your brain and body, and about attachment theory and how developing secure attachments can help you have healthy future relationships. Therapists who specialize in IPV, regardless of what treatment modality they use, can help you learn about these topics.

EYE MOVEMENT DESENSITIZATION AND REPROCESSING (EMDR)
As with other kinds of trauma, EMDR is a helpful form of therapy for people recovering from IPV. You can read more about EMDR on page 59.

Strategies to Try

USE ONLINE RESOURCES
The National Domestic Violence Hotline has a wealth of information for those looking to escape IPV, including resources available in your local community. If you worry about your partner finding out that you've been looking for support online, know that most of the major IPV support websites include an "escape" button you can click to quickly exit the website. However, these sites also warn that if you are worried about your emotional or physical safety, you should take additional steps such as clearing your browsing data.

FIND PEER SUPPORT
The IPV survivor community is vibrant and strong, and most local IPV/domestic violence centers have resources for peer-run support groups or peer counseling. Many survivors find it helpful to hear from others who have been through what they are currently experiencing.

SPEAK OPENLY WITH YOUR HEALTH CARE CLINICIAN
If you feel comfortable doing so, open up about your concerns to your health care clinicians, such as your primary care clinician or other medical clinician. The role of your health care clinician is to acknowledge the problem by having an open and nonjudgmental discussion about IPV. They can help you assess your safety, discuss the situation with you, encourage a strong safety plan, and refer you to local or national community resources.[5]

There are a handful of states in the US in which clinicians are mandated to report IPV-related injuries, or in general, significant injuries such as those caused by firearms. Otherwise, in most situations your confidentiality will be the top priority when discussing IPV. Ensure your comfort by asking your clinician in what circumstances they would need to report the information you share.

INTIMATE PARTNER VIOLENCE

Barriers to Escaping Intimate Partner Violence

THREATS TO YOUR SAFETY OR THE SAFETY OF OTHERS

IPV may involve threats to your own safety or the safety of your loved ones, particularly as a means to control you and keep you in the relationship. Additionally, your partner may have threatened to harm themselves if you were to leave. This could result in you feeling responsible for the safety of those you care about.

THE SLOW BOIL

Many survivors of IPV report that they didn't realize they were in an unhealthy relationship until it felt too late to leave. By that point, you may be isolated from supports or too financially dependent on the abuser to get out.

GASLIGHTING

Gaslighting is a tactic to make one feel as though they cannot trust their own perception, feelings, and decisions.[6] Your partner may say "You're being too emotional," or "You can't trust your friends. You know you're a bad judge of character."

Isolation from family and loved ones is often found within IPV. This is usually intentional on the part of the abuser, who isolates their partner from support systems in order to exert more control over them.

LACK OF UNDERSTANDING FROM COMMUNITY AGENCIES

For some communities, contacting the police after experiencing physical or sexual violence does not feel safe. In addition, going to authorities to file charges can be retraumatizing. Although this is not always the case, you may feel as though your experiences are being minimized, invalidated, or judged, or you may fear these things will happen after your partner, who has assumed a place of authority over you, has continually minimized the harm done. Also, you may find a lack of resources in your community for transportation or shelter when you are ready to leave the abusive relationship.

However, when you can connect to a helpful community agency, they can provide invaluable safety resources and support, including guiding you through whether you are eligible for a restraining order/Protection from Abuse order (PFA), and helping you with national programs such as the Address Confidentiality Program when needed.

THE EMOTIONAL IMPACT OF IPV

Many of our clients talk about feeling inadequate and shameful for both having experienced IPV and staying with the partner for as long as they did. Within the abusive relationship, you may have been made to feel small, inadequate, and that you are to blame for what's happening to you. Being in an abusive relationship can cause depression, anxiety, and Post-Traumatic Stress Disorder. These diagnoses can be challenging to navigate when in a healthy relationship, and even more challenging to manage in an abusive relationship.

THE DESIRE TO STICK WITH THE DEVIL YOU KNOW

As terrifying and harmful as IPV and unhealthy relationships are, sometimes it feels as though you don't know any other way of living, particularly if you've been in a long-term IPV relationship or have grown up in an abusive or toxic environment. There is a certain reliability in the instability. Leaving the relationship and walking into a new beginning can be scary and overwhelming.

Furthermore, if you have not been introduced to or seen a model of what a healthy relationship resembles, your frame of reference for what being loved looks like can be skewed by your exposure to unhealthy relationship dynamics. You may think, *I don't know how to be in a healthy relationship. What does that even look like?* For more information, see chapter 10.

THE RESEARCH SAYS . . .

You May Also Experience These Things

IPV can negatively impact physical and mental health, including increased chronic pain (page 198), gastrointestinal disorders, asthma, strokes, sexually transmitted diseases, alcohol and substance abuse (page 188), depression (page 8), Post-Traumatic Stress Disorder (page 57), and suicide.[7] Women who experience IPV, compared with those who don't, are more likely to engage in unhealthy behaviors and experience cardiovascular symptoms with long-term complications (likely due in part to the chronic stress of experiencing IPV).[8]

How to Communicate About Intimate Partner Violence

IF YOU'RE THE ONE EXPERIENCING IPV

Telling friends or family that you have been in an abusive relationship can be difficult. Many survivors report feeling shame and embarrassment. However, getting back that support is a crucial step toward breaking the cycle of isolation and abuse. No matter the response of your loved ones, it's still an important step to tell the people you trust so you can get the support you deserve.

If it feels too hard to tell them in person, consider writing a text message or an email. It's okay to set limits on the conversation, such as saying that you don't want them to ask questions about the abuse. Moreover, it's often helpful to tell them specifically how they can best support you. You might consider asking them for clothing donations, rides to IPV-related appointments or court, to help cook or to share a meal with you, and to remind you that you deserve healthy, loving relationships.

IF A LOVED ONE IS EXPERIENCING IPV

Some good words for us all to live by are "Remain curious, not judgmental." We all do the best we can with the information we have at the time. As an outsider in the relationship, you may have a bird's-eye view, but no one has a bird's-eye view of their own life, and hearing your input about what they could have done differently is not what a survivor of IPV needs. Instead, continue to be a healthy support, even if and when they go back to the abusive relationship. You are not supporting the abuse, you are supporting your loved one while also honoring your limits and boundaries. It is said that it takes an average of seven attempts for a person to leave an abusive relationship for good.

IF A CHILD HAS WITNESSED OR EXPERIENCED IPV

IPV doesn't only affect the person the violence is directed toward, but also those who are in the same space, which often includes children. A child's exposure can include witnessing or even just being aware of IPV, meaning the child does not have to see violence between caregivers for there to be a harmful impact.[9] Adolescents may also directly experience IPV in their early relationships.

Because witnessing IPV is one of the Adverse Childhood Experiences researched in the ACE study discussed on page 68, chapter 7 has many resources to consider for children confronted by IPV. Trauma-specific therapy may be helpful. One such therapy is Trauma-Focused Cognitive Behavioral Therapy (TF-CBT), which we discuss on pages 60 and 150.[10] You may worry about your children not having the same quality of life after a divorce or breakup. However, you may also feel guilty that you did not leave sooner. If you are a parent who has survived IPV, we want you to hear us on this: You did the best that you could with the resources and information you had at the time.

What Dealing with Intimate Partner Violence Can Look Like in Real Life

There are many manifestations of IPV. Some of them include physical violence, and others do not. We are sharing a common presentation of a woman in a heterosexual relationship, but if you do not see yourself reflected in this case example, please know that does not mean your experience of IPV is not valid.

Amy thought she had met the man of her dreams when she met Greg. They quickly got married in the ceremony she'd always imagined. But it didn't take long for it all to unravel. On the last day of their honeymoon, she found herself in tears because he made her feel so bad about how she looked in her bathing suit. Greg apologized, saying it was the stress of the wedding that had gotten to him. Amy understood and was sure everything would get better once they were home.

Back home, Amy continued to notice Greg's quick temper and the way he wanted to control every decision. So slowly she thought she was imagining it, things got worse. Greg told her he didn't like her hanging out with her friends. When she argued, he told her he wanted all of her time to himself. Amy relented, thinking it was only natural for newlyweds to spend all their time together.

They'd been married six months when Amy realized the only person she ever saw anymore was Greg. When she brought up going back to work, Greg told her how perfect it was to have her at home. He stopped letting her open the bills, saying that since he made all the money, he would worry about it.

Amy and Greg hadn't even been married a year when she found out she was pregnant. She was shocked because they'd been using condoms. Greg had told her not to take birth control because he didn't want her acting "crazy." Amy couldn't shake the feeling that this wasn't supposed to happen. And now Greg's behavior got even worse, telling her all the reasons she would be a bad parent, and even saying that she'd gotten so fat during pregnancy that he didn't have a choice but to have sex with other women. At an appointment with her ob-gyn, she broke down crying, and the clinician gave her a pamphlet for a local women's center.

The next week, when she knew Greg was at work, Amy went to the free group at the women's center. The group facilitator explained the Power and Control Wheel, and Amy recognized the tactics Greg had used. She learned that what had happened to her was part of the dynamic of an abusive relationship, and that isolating a person from their friends and family, keeping them from work, and having total control of the finances are common in relationships with IPV. She realized that there is even a name for when a partner deliberately gets you pregnant to have you more under their control: "stealthing."

The group facilitator suggested that Amy try some individual counseling sessions. As she talked to her counselor about her history of being bullied in middle school and a series of cheating boyfriends in college, she realized her self-esteem had taken a blow, which had made her vulnerable to staying with Greg. Looking at these patterns was hard, but Amy was committed to healing her self-esteem, so it wouldn't impact any future relationships, or her relationship with her baby. After coming to these realizations, she made the decision to leave Greg, and with the help of her support system, she did leave him.

The National Domestic Violence Hotline has advocates who are available 24-7 to give you support and help you find local resources. Call 1-800-799-7233, text 88788, or use the website's chat feature at thehotline.org. Access more information about online safety for victims of IPV at thehotline.org, a program of the National Domestic Violence Hotline.

READING LIST AND OTHER RESOURCES

Local YWCAs often have programs for people and families who have experienced IPV. Reach out to your local YWCA to see what they offer.

The National Center on Domestic Violence, Trauma, and Mental Health offers research and training for those looking to understand IPV and help prevent it.

Those looking for more resources to stay safe online can check out the National Network to End Domestic Violence (NNEDV)'s Safety Net Project's website, at nnedv.org.

The Black Woman's Guide to Overcoming Domestic Violence: Tools to Move Beyond Trauma, Reclaim Freedom, and Create the Life You Deserve by Robyn Gobin and Shavonne J. Moore-Lobban is an excellent guide to healing from the impact of IPV, and especially aims to support Black women.

The Violence is a fictional book by Delilah S. Dawson, whose mother was a survivor of IPV. Some survivors have found this dystopian revenge fantasy to be a cathartic read, and it can help the loved ones of IPV survivors understand what coercion and control feel like. However, this book is not for every survivor, as some of the content can be distressing.

Maid is a miniseries based on Stephanie Land's memoir *Maid: Hard Work, Low Pay, and a Mother's Will to Survive*. It highlights the challenges in recognizing that you are experiencing IPV, and the steps potentially needed to leave the relationship, as well as the emotional and psychological impact of IPV and generational trauma. (Note that it shows depictions of physical and emotional abuse.)

For more resources, see the lists on pages 66 and 111.

16

4

PHYSICAL HEALTH

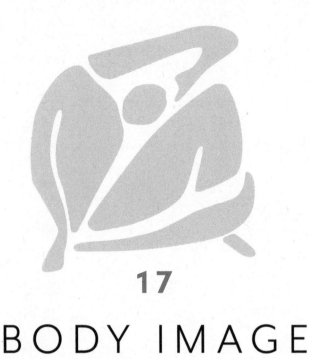

17

BODY IMAGE

W e all have bodies. Our bodies are all different shapes, sizes, and colors, with different levels of ability. One of the most marvelous things about being a human is that we get to experience the world in a body, likely using senses such as smell and taste. However, we also live in a world where some bodies are valued more than others due to racism, ableism, and capitalism.

"Body image" refers to the thoughts and feelings you have about your physical appearance, and how those thoughts and feelings cause you to behave. If you have a poor body image due to societal messages, your thoughts about your body may be unhelpful or negative, or you may have feelings of shame or disgust. These thoughts and feelings can lead to social isolation, disordered eating, use of addictive or harmful substances such as steroids or diet pills, and more.

Because of how your brain works, which scientists call "neuroplasticity,"[1] these behaviors can create feedback loops in which the behaviors reinforce the thoughts, and so on. For example, when you think and feel bad about your body, you're less likely to exercise.

However, moving your body in ways you enjoy and within your ability can help you feel better, not because of weight or appearance but because it can help you think about and appreciate how your body functions for you.[2] What if you could get out of the feedback loop that keeps you stuck in unhelpful body-related thoughts and behaviors, and find a new way to have a relationship with your body?

What Professional Help Can Look Like

Cognitive Behavioral Therapy (CBT) can help you manage and shift the thoughts that underlie the feelings and behaviors you experience.[3] If you can shift how you think about your body, you can change how you feel, and then how you behave. It is helpful to recognize when you engage in unhelpful thinking habits, as these may add to your tendency to compare yourself negatively to others.

Strategies to Try

USE AFFIRMATIONS

Even if you don't currently have access to professional therapy, there are many CBT strategies you can use yourself, including practicing self-compassion, which is an effective tool for increasing body appreciation.[4] One way to start is with affirmations.

You may have wondered if affirmations seem a little too fluffy. Could something so basic possibly work? However, research supports the idea that affirmations help us change our thoughts, especially if those affirmations are about our intrinsic qualities instead of our external ones.[5] For example, using affirmations like "I trust the wisdom of my body," or "My body deserves love," would be more helpful than affirmations focusing specifically on physical characteristics.

Research has found that appreciating your body leads to overall feelings of well-being, but if "body love" or "body positivity" feel too difficult to attain, you can instead try focusing on "body acceptance" or "body neutrality." Some body-neutral affirmations may include "My body is for living, not looking," or "The way my body looks is the least interesting thing about me."

It's important not to use affirmations to avoid difficult emotions. Affirmations are meant to be something you practice for the health of your brain, not a way to avoid things that don't feel good.

Use shower crayons to write affirmations on the walls of the shower or bathtub! Since shower crayons are harder to clean off the longer you leave them on, it's a good incentive to change your affirmation every few days.

SEEK OUT BODY POSITIVITY OR BODY NEUTRALITY

Follow social media accounts and other media that portray a diversity of body types in a positive or neutral light and surround yourself with people who appreciate their bodies despite perceived flaws. Our social context, including friends and romantic partners, matters when it comes to how we perceive our bodies, so exposing ourselves to body-positive social media can help.[7]

TREAT YOUR BODY AS YOU WOULD TREAT A LOVED ONE

The term "self-care" may be overused, but at its root it means to care for this one and only self you've been given to move through the world with, and that includes your body. See if you can make befriending your body a goal. We usually make friends slowly, over a period of intentional time and effort. Treating your body with small acts of kindness—stretching when you've been sitting for long periods of time, keeping it hydrated, going for regular check-ups, and treating it to a bath or your favorite food—communicates to your body that it's worth being cared for.

Try saying "thank you" to it during these acts, to make even the smallest daily habits like taking a walk or eating a nourishing meal an act of intentional self-care.

Barriers to Healing Your Body Image

Barriers to loving or accepting our bodies are all around us. Cultural norms, capitalism, ableism, racism, the patriarchy, and homophobia are only a few of the challenges you may face when trying to accept and love your body as it is. We are inundated with photoshopped, unrealistic images of bodies, and with messages trying to convince us to buy products or services to make our bodies look more like the ones we see in the media. According to research, if you can think critically about these messages (instead of accepting what they present as desirable or the norm), you will have a better body image.[8]

ABLEISM

Our culture of ableism, which puts a high priority on what the human body can do, can be a barrier to anyone who is impacted by injury, chronic illness, disability, or anything else that impedes the body's ability to move easily through the world, including aging.

People who advocate for disability rights say that it is not the disability that contributes to the negative body image, but the culture of ableism that surrounds us all. We can all become advocates for abolishing ableism, which will not only positively impact the community of people with disabilities, but all of us when we inevitably face body challenges due to injury, illness, or aging.

BODY DYSMORPHIA

Body dysmorphia can affect anyone, but people in the transgender community in particular may experience it before transitioning (whether the transition is physical, social, or other), and they may experience increased self-criticism and social distress related to their bodies before they are able to consolidate their gender identity.[9] People who identify as LGBTQ+ also often report that the way their bodies do or do not fit into cultural norms is a matter of their physical, emotional, and relational safety, similar to how it is for Black, Indigenous, and Asian people, or other racial minorities in the US.[10]

UNREALISTIC STANDARDS

It bears repeating that one of the biggest barriers to healthy body image are the unrealistic standards that surround us. Because of this, body neutrality often becomes the goal to work toward; it can often feel impossible in today's world to think positively about our bodies.

Body neutrality is a good step toward body appreciation, and it may be where you are most comfortable landing. The research, however, suggests that eventually focusing on appreciating, respecting, honoring, and even celebrating our bodies will help us move toward a healthier body image.[11]

How to Communicate About Your Body Image

IF YOU'RE THE ONE WITH POOR BODY IMAGE

If you can, be honest about your experiences with someone who is emotionally safe. Often, people dealing with poor body image find that their loved ones are experiencing this, too. Instead of feeling alone, sharing your body image thoughts with a trusted loved one can help you feel connected and provide accountability for enacting some of the tips we've shared above.

IF A LOVED ONE HAS POOR BODY IMAGE

Ask them how they would prefer to be supported. Some people like to hear positive things about themselves on their journey to body acceptance or love. Others may find this uncomfortable. You won't know unless you ask, so consider having an honest conversation about what support looks like. Also remember how important our social context is when it comes to body image and try to notice how you're thinking and speaking about your own body. Whether positive or negative, it will have a direct impact on your loved one.

IF THE PERSON WITH POOR BODY IMAGE IS A CHILD

Think about how you can model behavior for them. If children hear you or other loved ones complain about your looks or make disparaging remarks about bodies, they will learn to do the same.

We don't share this to shame you or to demand perfection; instead, see it as an opportunity. If you are having a hard time speaking to and treating your body kindly, you may find it easier to do so when you consider the impact your body image has on your child. Imagine a world in which your child grows up thinking that all bodies are wonderful because they let us experience the world! That is possible, if you show them the way.

What Healing Your Body Image Can Look Like in Real Life

Lila had always struggled with a hate for her body, but for most of her life, she thought that was completely normal. After all, her mom hated her body and everyone on social media always seemed to be trying to change their shape. It wasn't until she got a serious medical diagnosis and was trying to figure out how to improve her body's health that she realized how damaging all those years of self-hate had been.

Lila decided to see a therapist, who taught her that changing our body image starts with changing our thoughts about our bodies, from those of self-hatred to self-compassion. The therapist helped her slowly build affirmations that she could believe. Lila started with "My body deserves my care." She set alarms on her phone to remind her of this several times a day, and she wrote it on sticky notes that she stuck on all of her mirrors. After a while of practicing this thought, it started to feel obvious. Her therapist told her that meant it was time to try a new thought, so Lila decided on "My body is a good body." She changed all of her alarms and sticky notes to this new affirmation, and she also added saying it to herself every time she washed her hands.

Her therapist let her know that the human brain is like a muscle—we have to work it out regularly with healthy thinking, but we also need to increase the challenge level every once in a while, to make sure it doesn't stagnate. Over time, these CBT thought-changing methods began to shift the way Lila thought about her body.

Additionally, her therapist encouraged her to use Eye Movement Desensitization and Reprocessing (EMDR) to process some of the old messages she had absorbed around bodies. Lila was able to recognize and release old patterns she had learned from her family, friends, and culture that had been keeping her stuck. She found herself beginning to appreciate all the things her body did for her every day, and finally, truly started treating it like a friend.

READING LIST AND OTHER RESOURCES

The Body Is Not an Apology: The Power of Radical Self-Love by Sonya Renee Taylor aims at dismantling the ways systems of oppression have shaped our views of our bodies. It's a revolutionary call to action both internally and externally.

The Wisdom of Your Body: Finding Healing, Wholeness, and Connection Through Embodied Living by Hillary L. McBride is a beautiful examination of what it can mean to be embodied despite the damage we and our bodies experience in the world.

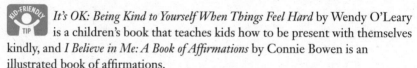 *It's OK: Being Kind to Yourself When Things Feel Hard* by Wendy O'Leary is a children's book that teaches kids how to be present with themselves kindly, and *I Believe in Me: A Book of Affirmations* by Connie Bowen is an illustrated book of affirmations.

The Body Liberation Project: How Understanding Racism and Diet Culture Helps Cultivate Joy and Build Collective Freedom by Chrissy King can help you understand the subconscious messages of racism and diet culture and move beyond them.

The Body Image Workbook: An Eight-Step Program for Learning to Like Your Looks by Thomas Cash provides education and worksheets on exploring and improving your perception of your body.

The Compassionate Mind by Paul Gilbert focuses on exploring the different systems in which you regulate your emotions, the impact they have on you, and how to utilize compassion to heal those imbalances in how you think about your body.

Every Body Yoga: Let Go of Fear, Get on The Mat, Love Your Body by Jessamyn Stanley can help if you want to move your body more but don't know if you can with your body shape, size, or ability. The author also offers online yoga resources.

Health At Every Size (asdah.org/health-at-every-size-haes-approach) is an organization centered on promoting health equity, ending weight-related discrimination, and advocating for accessible, quality care for persons of all body types.

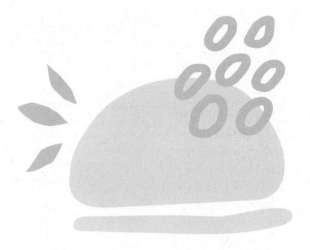

18

RELATIONSHIP
WITH FOOD

18

RELATIONSHIP WITH FOOD

ood is a source of life, however, it may be a source of distress or emotional coping for you. Having an unhealthy relationship with food may present itself in several ways. Binging is one avenue of this, when you eat more than one would typically eat in one sitting, feel as though you don't have the control to stop eating, and may experience intense guilt, shame, and frustration afterward.[1] This may be a standalone experience, although you may engage in excessive exercise, laxative use, vomiting, or not eating as much or at all at other meals to "compensate" for binging. In the other direction is intentionally restricting your food intake as a means of controlling your weight.[2] You may also excessively exercise or engage in other weight loss methods.

Control is a theme on both ends of the spectrum—whether you are feeling you lack control or are desperately looking to control, you end up in the same place: trying to satisfy something with unsatisfactory results. Guilt and shame are commonly experienced emotions in relationships with food, and may lead to isolation, secret eating, and increased negative self-talk.

You may be familiar with some eating disorders (ED), such as Anorexia Nervosa, Bulimia Nervosa, and Binge Eating Disorder, although there are others. Having an unhealthy relationship with food doesn't necessarily mean that you live with an eating disorder, similarly to how you can feel sad without being depressed. "Disordered eating" is often used to describe unhealthy eating patterns that don't presently warrant an ED diagnosis. To explore your relationship with food, reflect on the following questions. If you answer "yes" to any of them, you may benefit from improving your relationship with food, and your body.

- Does meal planning take up most of your day and mental space? Does it feel almost obsessive?

- Do you get anxious when food plans change?

- Do you have "safe" foods (foods that don't cause you anxiety to eat) or food rules?

- When you're presented with "unsafe" foods, do you feel panicked and out of control?

- Do you find that you eat little during the day and then eat to the point of being uncomfortably full or sick later on?

- Do you eat in secret, and would you feel shame if someone were to find out what you ate?

- Do you obsessively check your body in the mirror and pick it apart?

- Do you avoid looking at your body in the mirror, or at all?

- Do you feel that your weight, according to your scale, is your emotional barometer for the day?

- Do you find yourself obsessively focusing on healthy foods and clean eating and feel anxious around certain foods?

In this journey, it's important to keep in mind that healing is not linear; it is multidirectional. Feeling as though you are moving two steps forward, four steps back is not uncommon, and it is *not* failure. Each moment is an opportunity to show self-compassion and to be honest with yourself about what kind of support you need.

What Professional Help May Look Like

As you're healing your relationship with food, it can be helpful to have a team of clinicians to assist you in this journey. This may look like meeting with a dietitian, a therapist (to build skills to manage emotions and reframe thoughts), and your primary care clinician (to ensure your body is functioning in the way it needs).

MEETING WITH A DIETITIAN
A dietitian can help you build a healthier relationship with food by identifying what works for your body and what adequate nourishment looks like. If you are experiencing restricting or binging, make sure that the dietitian specializes in eating disorders.

COGNITIVE BEHAVIOR THERAPY FOR EATING DISORDERS
Cognitive Behavior Therapy for Eating Disorders (CBT-E) includes interventions to address over-evaluation (constantly judging and scrutinizing) of your body shape and weight.[7] This can include focusing on self-esteem, clinical perfectionism (having unrealistic expectations of yourself and intense self-criticism that often leads to depression and anxiety), and interpersonal problems, which often fuel and maintain disordered eating. CBT-E can also aid in challenging food rules (for example, "I can only eat these specific foods") and cognitive rigidity (seeing things in black and white and having trouble with the in-between), which maintain unhealthy eating patterns, poor self-concept, and barriers to positive behavior change.

COMPASSION-FOCUSED THERAPY FOR EATING DISORDERS
To address the higher levels of self-criticism and shame and the lower levels of self-compassion often associated with eating and weight concerns there is Compassion-Focused Therapy for Eating Disorders (CFT-E).[8]

CFT-E helps you develop understanding and acceptance of your body and its need for nutrition, activity, and rest.[9]

FAMILY-BASED THERAPY FOR EATING DISORDERS

Research says that parents should also be involved in eating disorder treatment for children. In particular, the research has identified Family-Based Therapy as the most helpful approach for kids who have eating disorders.[10] It focuses on educating the family without blame and engaging them all in healthy eating habits.[11]

Strategies to Try

PRACTICE MINDFULNESS WHILE EATING

Mindfulness is a helpful practice when it comes to building a healthier relationship with food, and also with your thoughts and emotions. This includes being mindful of what and how you eat, but also how you think about food. "I earned breakfast" may be an innocent statement for some, although for others, it may promote the belief that food in general or certain foods need to be "earned." Similarly, statements such as "Ugh, I'm going to have to go to the gym to work this off" promote widespread unhealthy beliefs around "treating ourselves."

Be mindful of what you're doing when you are eating, such as working or doomscrolling on your phone. These activities may serve to distract you from eating, so you may not notice when you are getting full. Focusing on eating can help you set and maintain healthy habits around your relationship with food. You may benefit from the strategy of placing your fork

> **THE RESEARCH SAYS . . .**
>
> ### This Is What's Happening In Your Brain and Body
>
> You may experience disruptions in your natural hunger and fullness cues if you engage in binging or restricting, as they are often ignored or become distorted. With restricting, hunger cues are ignored as you may fear gaining weight, and when you do eat, you are not necessarily eating to fullness. With binging, emotional hunger often gets confused with physical hunger, and you may not notice or may find listening to your fullness cues near impossible. You may feel largely disconnected from your body, while feeling overly aware of your body at other times.

down between each bite to give yourself time to fully chew and savor your food, which can also lead to increased enjoyment of the meal.

If being mindful for a whole meal feels like too big of a goal, try practicing with something smaller, like a Hershey's Kiss. Before you even get to the chocolate, notice the color and texture of the foil it's wrapped in. Be mindful of the crinkling sound the foil makes. Then notice how the chocolate looks and smells. Finally, take your time to let it slowly melt on your tongue, savoring the taste. Practicing mindfulness in small ways like this can teach you how to be present with food.

 MINDFUL EATING FOR KIDS
If you eat meals as a family, consider taking turns to mindfully describe and enjoy each item on the table.

CHECK IN WITH YOUR MOOD

Having a challenging time managing or experiencing your emotions may lead you to using food as a means of coping or avoidance. Check in with how you're feeling prior to, during, or after a meal. This can look like taking three deep breaths to settle in, then writing down any emotions and thoughts that arise. It can be helpful to set a reminder on your phone or have a sticky note next to the place you normally eat. If it feels overwhelming to do a mood check around a meal, instead consider practicing in the morning or night by checking in with how you're feeling.

If you check out during meals, you may be eating so quickly that your body doesn't have a chance to register its fullness cues. Set the intention to slow down. This can mean slowly chewing your food, noticing its texture and taste. Doing this for your entire meal may not feel possible at first, and that's okay. You can start by slowing down for one bite and gradually increasing the number of bites as you feel able. Next, see if you can notice your emotional response to the food, and any thoughts you are having about it.

ESTABLISH REGULAR TIMES FOR EATING

In general, not eating enough can make you feel lethargic, less able to concentrate, and more irritable. Skipping a meal or not eating enough may increase your risk of binging later. It can be helpful to have regular time frames for meals, and to have snacks available if you get hungry in between.

CHANGE YOUR RELATIONSHIP WITH EXERCISE

If you are hyperfocused on exercise as a means of weight loss, one strategy is to recognize the other benefits of exercise. You may find that it clears your mind, gives you energy, and helps you feel strong. Before and while you exercise, be sure to point this out to yourself.

You can also consider conscious movement, which is not about burning calories or increasing your heart rate, it's about slowing down, connecting with your body in positive ways, and giving space for your mind to relax as well. It can be a healthier approach if you are not properly nourishing your body. Intense exercise and improper nourishment can lead to cardiac issues, dehydration, and disruptions in your body's ability to heal and recover.[12]

 When talking to kids about exercise, frame it as a way to help keep their joints, muscles, and bones healthy, and to have fun together.

SELF-VALIDATION

If you struggle with nourishing your body or with negative body image (check out chapter 17), it can be helpful to have positive self-statements written on a Post-it note or in your phone for you to access as you need. These could be "It is okay for me to nourish my body," or "My body deserves to be treated well." You could keep these notes in your bedroom (as you're picking out your clothes for the day), on your mirror (where you may be engaging in body checking or negative body-image comments), on your refrigerator or microwave, or where you typically eat.

Barriers to Healing Your Relationship with Food

DIET CULTURE, FAMILY DYNAMICS, AND SOCIETAL PRESSURES

Growing up in a society that applauds smaller bodies and essentially avoids all other body types doesn't exactly foster positive body image. In addition, many who experience food challenges have grown up in families in which negative feelings about food and body image have been passed down.

If you have a relative who has made negative comments about their own bodies ("Ugh, I look horrible"), the amount of food that they ate ("I can't believe I ate that much, I'm going to have to exercise for days to make up for it"), or who you've witnessed go on many diets, chances are their words and actions have taught you that this is the way you're supposed to treat your body.

You may know people who've made critical comments about your eating habits or body, contributing to or worsening your perception of your body and food. Unfortunately, people are notorious for commenting on our bodies when it's none of their business.

There are other times when your loved ones may share their concerns, as they may notice a problem building before you do. Sometimes, this can open the door for you to begin your healing process, although it could potentially be delivered in an unsupportive way or at a time when you are not ready to hear it, which could lead you to withdraw, and increase your feelings of shame.

NEGATIVE COMPARISONS ON SOCIAL MEDIA

Social media can be a source of misinformation, misrepresentation, and negative comparison to others. Pro–eating disorder content is rampant online, such as encouragement to severely restrict your food in order to lose weight. Additionally, some photo filters and other editing tools have created an unrealistic portrayal of bodies.

As we discuss in chapter 17, intentionally following social media influencers of all sizes and shapes, or advocates of the Health at Every Size movement, can help transform your social media experience.

FAT PHOBIA AND ASSUMPTIONS ABOUT BODY SIZE

Many people believe that if you have a smaller body, you are inherently healthier and have more worth, and if you have a larger body, then you are unhealthy and have less worth. This is absolutely not true.

As for health, you can be any body size and potentially fall anywhere on the spectrum of great to problematic health. It's also important to recognize that we all have different metabolisms. The societal and individual judgments placed on those in larger bodies—that they are at fault for their body size, that they are failing in some way, or that they are morally wrong—has profound negative emotional, mental, and physical impacts.

THE NEGATIVE PHYSICAL IMPACTS OF DISORDERED EATING

There is the potential for serious negative impact on your body through restricting, binging, laxative abuse, intentional vomiting, and yo-yo dieting. It can be challenging to manage the emotional and mental struggles of disordered eating while also coping with the physical impacts, such as gastrointestinal problems, damage to your teeth enamel, and decreases in bone density. If your relationship with food has reached an extremely unhealthy place, it may require a team of medical clinicians to help you manage all of these impacts.

FEELING INVALIDATED BY PROFESSIONALS WHO DON'T UNDERSTAND

THE RESEARCH SAYS . . .

You May Also Experience These Things

People living with eating disorders often experience anxiety (page 19), perfectionism, depression (page 8), and trauma and Post-Traumatic Stress Disorder (page 57); this may proceed ED experiences, or ED experiences may be in response to mental health challenges.[13] People with Polycystic Ovary Syndrome are also more likely to have an unhealthy relationship with their food and weight.[14]

You may have felt judged or invalidated by a mental health or medical professional who was meant to help you. Many of our clients have shared that they were fearful of seeing a clinician after receiving hurtful comments about their weight from other professionals or dealing with clinicians who lack experience in disordered eating.

We encourage you to advocate for yourself by expressing your thoughts about the breakdown in communication and remember that it is well within your rights to seek care from a new clinician. (For more, see chapters 24 and 25.) If you are being seen in a group practice, you may be able to request a clinician reassignment.

UNHEALTHY VALIDATION FROM OTHERS

In the course of unhealthy dieting, or eating less than what your body truly needs, and other unhelpful eating-related behaviors, you may end up receiving validation from others for the shape of your body or for your food choices. While that validation can feel good, it can further encourage these unhealthy habits.

LACKING HEALTHY COPING SKILLS FOR MANAGING EMOTIONS

You may use food to shut down or avoid your emotions, but this provides only temporary relief. Inevitably, your emotions will come out and then you'll be dealing with the buildup of all the feelings that haven't been properly processed. Using outlets such as journaling, sharing your feelings with others, breathing techniques, as well as other strategies, may help you to recognize and share space with your emotions. At first this may be uncomfortable, but with time you will be able to learn to tolerate them. It's like lifting weights: Start small and build gradually.

How to Communicate about Your Relationship with Food

IF YOU'RE THE ONE EXPERIENCING CHALLENGES WITH FOOD

Educating others about what you need can be both an empowering and exhausting experience. When safe to do so, it is important to vocalize your needs and boundaries. You may consider saying, "Please do not make any comments about my body or what I'm eating." Or "When you make negative comments about your body, I worry that you're also having negative thoughts about my body. Let's set the intention to talk more positively about our bodies. Maybe we can even gently point out when we're noticing the other being unkind to themselves?"

IF A LOVED ONE IS EXPERIENCING CHALLENGES WITH FOOD

Reflect on your own relationship with food and your body, as well as how you talk about these areas to yourself and with others. How you talk about your own body and food may be activating to others, and it may either create distance or greater connection depending on how you navigate these topics. Being more mindful may be a way to show your loved one that you're thinking of them and their struggles.

Ask your loved one how they want to be supported and see if they want you to check in on their progress. They may need more support during the holiday season or summer, when there tends to be more social events with food and diet talk.

Consider using validating statements like "You are worthy of self-care, and I'll help you in any way that I can" or "I may not completely understand your struggle, although I imagine it's challenging. You don't get a break from food; it's something you have to confront each day. I see you, and I see your strength."

IF THE PERSON EXPERIENCING CHALLENGES WITH FOOD IS A CHILD

Discovering their food likes and dislikes is part of a child's discovery of the world. While they can be notoriously picky eaters, children can have a lot of variation in their relationships with food and still be well within the normal range. However, because most disordered eating develops by adolescence,[15] it's also important to keep an eye on things and seek professional intervention if your child is starting to engage in disordered eating. This can look like food avoidance, leaving immediately after meals, or irritability around certain foods.

Early intervention is associated with better rates of recovery, so if your child does need professional help, it's important to get it sooner rather than later.[16]

What Healing from an Eating Disorder Can Look Like in Real Life

Dan is feeling stressed and overwhelmed with work, and he doesn't feel like he has time for himself. He starts noticing that he's eating more than he usually does at night. It's comforting and it feels like the only activity that's completely his. Gradually, he finds that he is eating more in one sitting, and it's only during this time that he feels he can disengage from stress.

Dan's eating is starting to feel out of his control. He's not always noticing when he's full, and even if he does notice it, it feels like he can't stop. Once he does, he feels uncomfortably full, and sometimes experiences nausea or stomach pain. He feels so much shame around his eating habits; although, at the same time, it's the only source of relief—for a few minutes at least—that he seems to get in the day.

After months of this, Dan decides to meet with an eating disorder therapist. He talks at length about his relationship with food, as well as his family's relationship with food and how they talked about their bodies. He realizes that his mom talked negatively about her body and would often be on a diet. There was a lot of talk about "good" and "bad" foods, which created confusion for Dan once he had the freedom to make his own food choices. He learns that this is a common struggle for individuals who've had unhealthy models for food and body image.

Dan also learns that he struggles with responding to his emotions in healthy ways and to build coping skills to recognize and respond to what he's feeling rather than using food as a coping tool. He starts working with a dietitian to help create a meal plan to appropriately nourish his body. He has a team of trusted professionals to help him navigate building a healthier relationship with food. He starts to challenge some of the food rules he didn't even realize he'd created over the years. It's hard, and uncomfortable. He is unlearning a lifetime of negative thoughts and habits.

Over time, making food choices gets easier. Dan doesn't feel guilt or shame for eating those "bad" foods. He can look at himself in the mirror and smile, rather than tear himself apart. There are still some hard days, although they don't seem to linger as long as they did before. Dan learns to forgive himself, to be kind to himself, and to learn his patterns rather than shame himself. He didn't realize how much time was taken up thinking about food until now. He feels empowered. Food isn't the enemy anymore.

READING LIST AND OTHER RESOURCES

Brave Girl Eating: A Family's Struggle with Anorexia by Harriet Brown shares the impact of an eating disorder not only on the person with the disorder, but also the ripple effect that takes place within the family.

Life Without Ed: How One Woman Declared Independence from her Eating Disorder and You Can Too by Jenni Schaefer is a raw telling of a woman's struggle with an eating disorder and how she learned to gain back her independence and more importantly, herself.

Reclaiming Body Trust: A Path to Healing and Liberation by Hilary Kinavey and Dana Sturtevant is a beautiful book on how to break free from societal norms and truly find a home in your body.

Anti-Diet: Reclaim Your Time, Money, Well-Being, and Happiness Through Intuitive Eating by Christy Harrison, MPH, RD, is a book that sheds light on the toxic diet culture present in our society.

Physical is a television show depicting a woman's struggle with binge eating disorder and exercise addiction. The show has graphic depictions so you may want to proceed with caution, but it can also provide validation of how difficult the journey of eating disorder recovery can be.

For more resources, see page 176.

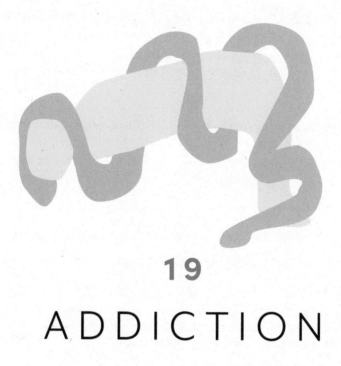

19

ADDICTION

I f you have struggled with addiction, it can seem impossible to recover, find compassionate treatment that works, or repair the damage you may have experienced in all areas of your life. There are many reasons, as varied as people are themselves, that may bring you to the use of a substance. At the same time, underneath many addictions is the common theme of trying to cope with or escape something that feels otherwise unmanageable.[1]

The use of substances can result in your engaging in problematic behaviors and can have negative consequences on your health, relationships, and occupational functioning. Substance use also puts you at risk for other mental health conditions, including suicidality. Alcohol use can increase unhealthy coping behaviors and hinder self-regulation, while opioid use can cause neurobiological changes that lead to increases in negative moods, and both create increased risk for suicidality.[2] You can find out more about the link between substance use and mental health crises, as well as what to do if you are experiencing one, in chapter 23.

Substances include alcohol, caffeine, cannabis (marijuana), hallucinogens, inhalants, opioids, sedatives/hypnotics/anxiolytics, stimulants, and tobacco.[3] Each category of substance is as unique as some of the symptoms they cause, but there is overlap in the diagnosis of their related "disorder," "intoxication," or "withdrawal."[4] Gambling is also considered a serious addiction.

Many substances have a related "use disorder" (for example, Tobacco Use Disorder) that include common criteria, though these may vary depending on the substance being used.[5] "Use disorder" refers to the point in which you are experiencing significant impairment in your life as a result of the substance(s) you are consuming. Addiction, which is often viewed as a severe "use disorder," is a chronic disorder that includes compulsive drug seeking, continued use of the substance(s) despite the consequences of doing so, and can result in long-term or irreversible negative changes within the brain.[6] By the time substance use has turned into an addiction, you may feel helpless to change the behavior. For example, 80 percent of cigarette smokers report wanting to quit smoking, and yet only 45 percent are eventually able to do so.[7] If you have been using substances for much of your life in a way that seems "normal" or socially acceptable, you may be surprised to find that you could still meet the criteria for a substance use disorder. For example, here are some of the diagnostic criteria for Alcohol Use Disorder,[8] which repeated studies have shown is increasing in the United States, especially among women.[9]

- A problematic pattern of alcohol use leading to clinically significant impairment or distress. This could include drinking more than intended, being unable to cut back on drinking, craving alcohol, spending a lot of time recovering from alcohol use, changing social or work activities due to alcohol use, and continuing to drink despite issues at work, in relationships, or being in dangerous situations.

- Tolerance, or the need for markedly increased amounts of alcohol to achieve intoxication or desired effect, or a markedly diminished effect with continued use of the same amount of alcohol.

- Withdrawal, in which stopping or reducing alcohol use that has been heavy and prolonged results in symptoms such as insomnia, increased hand tremors, anxiety, or nausea. You may experience additional symptoms of withdrawal and it may result in continued alcohol or substance use to avoid those symptoms.

Please note that given the number of substances and evolving treatments, this chapter is not exhaustive. We do hope it provides you with a good starting point for where to look for support.

What Professional Help May Look Like

A combination of psychosocial therapy and medications are helpful for the treatment of addiction, though the specific medication used in different studies varies.[11]

Research is clear that for treatment to be effective, it needs to be personalized to your biopsychosocial needs. This should include Trauma-Informed Care, shared decision-making, and a strong therapeutic alliance, meaning a safe and trusting relationship with your therapist.[12] As we stress in chapter 24, you are entitled to advocate for yourself if the care you are receiving is not what you need.

There are a variety of treatment settings for those recovering from substance use disorder, depending on the level of severity and potential for acute withdrawal symptoms. It is possible to receive all of your treatments in an outpatient setting, although depending on your needs, a detox or residential setting may be recommended (see also chapter 22).

MEDICATION-ASSISTED THERAPY

A front-line treatment for addiction is Medication-Assisted Therapy that combines the use of medication

THE RESEARCH SAYS . . .

This Is What's Happening in Your Brain and Body

Addiction affects neurocircuitry in the brain involved in reward and motivation, executive control, and emotional processing.[13] Substance use negatively impacts your ability to prioritize behaviors that result in long-term benefit rather than short-term rewards, even when associated with catastrophic consequences.[14] This means you seek immediate gratification driven by substances rather than the delayed gratification of stability.

such as methadone, buprenorphine, or naltrexone with counseling and behavioral therapies.[15] Sometimes, such treatment can be offered in your primary care office.

COGNITIVE BEHAVIORAL THERAPY
Cognitive Behavioral Therapy can help you identify the stressors that lead you to use substances and find more appropriate coping options.[16]

EYE MOVEMENT DESENSITIZATION AND REPROCESSING
Trauma therapy such as Eye Movement Desensitization and Reprocessing (EMDR) is often helpful to treat the root of your addiction, an important starting point so you do not replace one addiction with another. We also know from the ACE study (discussed in chapter 7) that you are more likely to develop addiction if you had childhood experiences of trauma.[17]

Addiction-focused EMDR targets the addiction behaviors and the trauma memories that may underlie them.[18] Numerous studies indicate that recovering from a substance use disorder is more difficult if you also have Post-Traumatic Stress Disorder.[19]

FAMILY THERAPY
KID-FRIENDLY TIP "People, places, and things" is the conventional wisdom within the twelve-step world, reminding us that if our environment does not change, we won't change either. Family therapy can help with this. Such treatment is also an important part of helping a child with their substance use disorder, as children are meant to be a part of a bigger attachment system.

Insecure attachment is one of the factors that leads to substance use in childhood and adolescence, and yet attachment can be repaired when the family is willing to come together, such as with Attachment-Based Family Therapy.[20]

Strategies to Try

JOIN A TWELVE-STEP FACILITATION TREATMENT
Twelve-step facilitation treatments, also known as twelve-step programs, can help you become engaged in a widely available, community-based, free, long-term recovery program aimed at keeping you in remission.[21]

In the United States, twelve-step support groups are highly accessible and can generally be found at any time of the day or night, if not in person in your local area then online. This has made them an invaluable resource. Twelve-step programs are usually peer run, which means that you will be learning from others who have experienced similar addiction issues, and may not have support from a licensed professional in the meeting. Twelve-step programs often have workbooks or "steps" that are meant to be worked at alongside attending the meetings. Our clients usually report the most success when they fully "work" the program, meaning that they complete the steps rather than only attending the meetings.

Many twelve-step programs encourage the use of a "sponsor," a peer with more experience maintaining sobriety, with whom you can connect personally for support and accountability. Soc ial support is an important part of recovery,[22] and for many people that support is found in twelve-step programs.

Every twelve-step group is different. If the first one or two you attend are not the right fit for you, keep trying! You will likely find a better fit and community that can help you through addiction recovery.

LOOK INTO HARM REDUCTION OPTIONS

Twelve-step and similar programs tend to promote an abstinence-only approach to substance use. This means that you aren't allowed to use alcohol or substances (often excluding nicotine or caffeine). You may find this difficult, and it may cause you to disengage in such treatment. However, there is another evidence-based approach to substance use treatment called "harm reduction."

Harm reduction aims to align with the desire that some people may have to reduce or control, but not completely discontinue, their substance use. Organizations such as the Food and Drug Administration and the American Psychiatric Association have begun to look at reduction in substance use as a desired goal instead of complete abstinence as the only standard.[23] Harm reduction can include strategies such as safe needle exchanges, distribution of overdose reversal medications, considering relapse as a typical part of recovery, and the use of Medication-Assisted Therapy (such as the use of buprenorphine or methadone).

Barriers to Getting Help for Addiction

According to the Substance Abuse and Mental Health Services Administration, the barriers to getting help that people with addiction report are as follows.[24]

NOT BEING READY TO STOP USING

About 39 percent of respondents said they were not ready to stop using. This is often the case when the existing factors that led you to addiction not only still exist, but perhaps have worsened throughout your addiction.

NOT KNOWING WHERE TO FIND TREATMENT

About 23 percent of respondents said they did not know where to go to find treatment, which is not surprising when you consider that less than 1 percent of the US's medical doctors specialize in addiction.[25] Additional barriers include lack of or insufficient insurance coverage (addiction treatment is typically not covered by insurance) and clinician availability. Based on 2012 data, it's estimated that thirty million people live in US counties without a single prescriber of buprenorphine treatment.[26] Since the COVID-19 pandemic, strides are being made to provide treatment and prescribe via telemedicine, but there is still a long way to go.[27]

THE STIGMA OF ADDICTION

Stigma exists in all corners of addiction, from the addiction itself to its treatment. If you've experienced addiction, you know firsthand how stigmatizing it is. About 17 percent of respondents said they did not seek help because of worry it might cause neighbors or the community to judge them, and about 16 percent worried it might have a negative effect on employment. Stigma associated with the medications for treating substance use disorder, such as methadone and buprenorphine, is related to the misconception that addiction is a willful choice, not a disease, as many hold the belief that recovery only exists in complete abstinence from all opioids.[28]

Stigma can become deeply internalized and anticipated, which may result in those with substance use struggles to avoid seeking care and subsequently experience poorer health outcomes.[29] The fear of stigma may result in you isolating yourself from others, and isolation can then directly drive an increase in substance use.[30]

RELAPSE

Relapse brings its own stigma and shame, although there is evidence that relapse is common at the beginning of substance use treatment, with some studies indicating 85 percent of people will relapse within their first year of treatment.[31] If you have experienced an addiction relapse, know that it is not the end of the road for you. Surround yourself with supportive people who will stay with you through your relapse. If you don't have access to those people personally, use the support of those who have shared their history of addiction and recovery publicly. You are worth the time, energy, and support it takes to walk a recovery journey.

THE RESEARCH SAYS . . .

You May Also Experience These Things

Having a Substance Use Disorder along with another mental health disorder such as depression (page 8), Bipolar Disorder, Borderline Personality Disorder (page 77) or Post-Traumatic Stress Disorder (page 57) is common, as many people turn to substances to cope with their other mental health concerns. This is called a dual diagnosis and can increase risk for suicidal behavior.[33] Relationship difficulties, job and financial stressors, recent heavy substance use, intoxication, a history of previous suicide attempts, and a history of sexual abuse may all compound the suicide risk for those with dual diagnoses.[34]

SYSTEMIC ISSUES

The systemic issues that people often face when recovering from addiction, including unemployment, criminal justice issues, and homelessness, can seem like insurmountable barriers.

Finding support can be a crucial part of overcoming these systemic issues.[32] This could be professional support, such as a drug and alcohol counselor, a case manager, or a peer support or recovery coach. You deserve the support you need to work through the aftermath of addiction.

How to Communicate About Addiction

IF YOU'RE THE ONE DEALING WITH ADDICTION

Feelings of guilt or shame may cause you to hesitate to speak openly to those around you. Remember that you are not alone in experiencing substance use. There are likely biological, psychological, and social factors making it difficult to change your behavior.

Ask others for help. Be honest with them about what you think will help you. It is common to experience lapses and relapses in substance use. Don't hide this fact but talk openly about what you feel set you back and problem solve how you can reduce the likelihood of relapse in the future.

If you are involved in treatment, seek out and speak openly with a therapist, clinician, and sponsor. People cannot support you if you avoid them.

IF A LOVED ONE IS DEALING WITH ADDICTION

Maintain a nonjudgmental stance. The substance use is the problem; your loved one is more than their substance use. It can be difficult to maintain compassion if you feel that your loved one has not been honest with you or has made unsafe decisions. We encourage you to maintain healthy boundaries and to say "no" when needed. When you are feeling able to provide support, ask open-ended questions (questions that start with "what" and "how") and listen patiently. Access resources, so that *you* can get some support during this process. With it, you will be more empowered and resourceful to support your loved one.

IF THE PERSON DEALING WITH ADDICTION IS A CHILD OR ADOLESCENT

Early intervention is key in preventing the addiction from becoming more severe.[35] The earlier the onset of general drug use is, including cannabis and alcohol, the more likely you are to develop an opioid or cocaine dependence later in life.[36]

Parental drug use is a factor in childhood substance use disorder onset,[37] so as with many topics covered in this book, making sure you are attending to your own sobriety will be an important part of helping your child.

If you discover that your child is using substances, your fear could lead you to panic and react in unhelpful ways. Sometimes parents go to the other extreme and support the substance use in order not to alienate the child. Try to remain curious and nonjudgmental about what could have led to the substance use, while also setting firm boundaries around the use itself.

What Getting Help for Addiction Can Look Like in Real Life

Charley mostly drank on the weekends, but over time the amount they drank went from two to three drinks a night to five to six. They started to notice they craved a drink by the end of the day and felt physically sick if they went too long without one.

They also started noticing increased trouble getting restful sleep at night. They didn't do it, but sometimes they considered having a beer in the mornings.

Charley talked to a friend who said Charley should cut back on how much they drink. The friend said that they had gone to their primary care clinician to be told that their Liver Function Tests (LFTs) showed damage to cells in their liver. They were told to cut back on their drinking and to be mindful of their diet. The friend thought Charley should do the same.

Charley felt skeptical about this advice but they knew how much their friend cared about them and so they agreed to get checked out.

The clinician talked to Charley about the risks of drinking multiple times a day, and about potential treatments, such as medication (like naltrexone), to help reduce and stop alcohol consumption. Charley was told that the clinician would need to work closely with them as withdrawal symptoms for alcohol can be dangerous. The clinician said Charley would have support every step of the way and informed them that they can and should go to the emergency room if they started to experience withdrawal.

Additionally, the clinician confirmed that it could be helpful to talk with someone to identify healthier coping strategies. Charley's therapist recommended a local twelve-step Alcoholics Anonymous (AA) group they could attend.

The first few times they went to the AA meeting, Charley felt worried about running into someone they knew. Soon though, they found themselves drawn in by the stories people told about their experiences getting sober. They heard themselves reflected in the stories. They began to feel less alone, and even spent time with the people from the meeting. They got a sponsor, and now when they need extra support they call their sponsor instead of having a beer.

A year into it, Charley gets their one-year sobriety chip. Looking back, they almost don't recognize themselves. They feel energetic and hopeful, and connected to a community that supports them living a healthy lifestyle. Charley knows recovery is a lifelong journey, but they also have the resources they need to continue.

Substance Abuse and Mental Health Services Administration (SAMHSA) has a free, confidential, 24-7 helpline that provides information, treatment referrals, support groups, and community-based organizations for those living with mental health and/or substance use disorders. The Helpline Number is 1-800-662-4357. They also have many online resources such as guides for family members at samhsa.gov/find-help/national-helpline.

READING LIST AND OTHER RESOURCES

The Many Lives of Mama Love: A Memoir of Lying, Stealing, Writing, and Healing by Lara Love Hardin addresses a heroin addiction that a middle-class mother never saw coming.

The Glass Castle by Jeannette Walls is a memoir that explores the impact of her parent's alcoholism on the family. The memoir also explores themes of child abuse, mental illness, and homelessness.

Demon Copperhead by Barbara Kingsolver is a novel that explores the route of addiction for a young man from the time he is born through young adulthood. If you are struggling to feel compassion for a loved one with addiction, this fictional work may help you understand the opioid crisis and its impact.

Adult Children of Alcoholics and Dysfunctional Families (adultchildren.org), previously known as Adult Children of Alcoholics, provides a twelve-step program for adults who grew up in households where they experienced abuse, neglect, and trauma, particularly as a result of a parent or parents struggling with alcoholism.

Al-Anon is a support system if you have a loved one struggling with alcohol use disorder. Go to al-anon.org.

Nar-Anon (nar-anon.org) is a support system if you have a loved one struggling with substance use disorder.

FindTreatment.gov is a confidential and anonymous resource if you are seeking treatment for mental and substance use disorders in the United States and its territories.

"Nuggets" is a five-minute YouTube video by Filmbilder & Friends that may provide some insight into the experiences of those with substance use disorders.

You may find it helpful to hear the personal stories of people who have recovered from addiction. Glennon Doyle's podcast *We Can Do Hard Things* and Dax Shepherd's podcast *Armchair Expert* offer a raw look at recovery as well as what life on the other side can look like.

19

ADDICTION

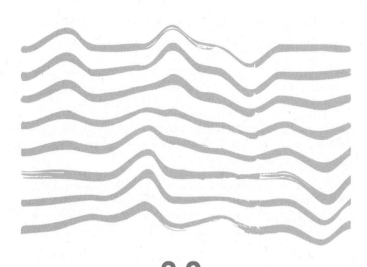

20

CHRONIC PAIN

C hronic pain can test your limits of endurance and directly impact your mental health, and yet many suffer daily from chronic pain that often seems to have no cure. Chronic pain is defined as pain that lasts beyond normal tissue healing time (around twelve weeks).[1] When functioning properly, pain is a way for us to recognize if we are in danger and need to take action. Sometimes our pain systems stop functioning as a warning and instead continually send us signals that something is wrong, even though there is no identifiable source for our pain. Common causes of chronic pain in older individuals include diabetic peripheral neuropathy, fibromyalgia, and osteoarthritis.[2]

How pain feels is unique to each person, and is influenced by biological, psychological, and social factors.[3] Your risk factors, like negative mood, and protective factors, such as your interpersonal relationships and coping skills, interact with your physical pain neurobiology to determine how you experience it.[4]

You are not at fault for your pain. Others may not understand how your pain impacts your functioning. Chronic pain may likely impede your activities of daily living, work and work efficiency, and reduce quality and quantity of life.[5] It can increase your likelihood of absenteeism, requests for changes in job duties, and loss of your job.[6] Read on to find out how the science can help you find a light in the darkness of chronic pain.

What Professional Help May Look Like

Treatments for chronic pain are most likely to be effective if they include some combination of prescribed medications, physical therapy, pain psychology interventions, social support from friends and family, and lifestyle changes.[7]

The first-line treatment for your chronic pain will depend on its cause. Of note, treatments such as surgery and injections are often not recommended as first-line treatments and if you are advised to consider these interventions, it's often most beneficial for them to be combined with less invasive treatments such as physical therapy, medication, mental health treatment such as talk therapy, and coping strategies.[8]

TALK THERAPY

Talk therapy does not follow a specific protocol, but gives you space each week to discuss what is uppermost on your mind, and could be helpful in managing your pain and finding support for the difficulty of living with it. However, such treatments remain underutilized, likely due to lack of awareness of their benefits and the difficulty in getting insurance coverage for such services.[9] Therapy for pain, particularly Cognitive Behavioral Therapy, Eye Movement Desensitization and Reprocessing, or Acceptance and Commitment Therapy may improve your levels of fatigue, sleep, depression, your quality of life, and work.[10]

With the help of your medical clinician, when treating your pain, you should consider psychosocial factors, including feelings of depression, anxiety, or fear, and your recovery expectations.[11] Speak with your medical clinician about how to consider all of these factors in setting realistic expectations for your pain and functional levels in the future.

COGNITIVE BEHAVIORAL THERAPY

Cognitive Behavioral Therapy (CBT) may help you cope with pain or related disabilities, or distress related to pain.[12] CBT for pain often includes relaxation training, coping strategies, exposure to feared activities, and activities that redirect attention from pain.[13]

Recognizing and challenging negative thoughts may be helpful in managing the catastrophic thinking that often comes with pain. For example, you may understandably think negative things like *My pain will continue to get worse. It will never improve.* CBT can help you find a new thought to practice, such as, "Instead of letting my pain control my life, today I am going to take a healthy step toward being in control."

EYE MOVEMENT DESENSITIZATION AND REPROCESSING

Eye Movement Desensitization and Reprocessing (EMDR) has been shown to be effective for resolving chronic pain,[14] especially when the pain has its origins in trauma or if it results in secondary trauma or stress.[15] In addition to processing the trauma either beneath or caused by the pain, EMDR can help you learn to communicate with your body and understand its needs.[16]

ACCEPTANCE AND COMMITMENT THERAPY

Acceptance and Commitment Therapy (ACT) may help you disengage from unsuccessful attempts to control or avoid pain, and instead move you toward pursuing goals and values more consistently.[17] ACT helps you be more psychologically flexible, open to experiences, to focus on your values, and maintain awareness of experiences in the present moment.[18]

MEDICATION

Some medications may be more helpful than others depending on the source of your pain. They may include things such as acetaminophen, non-steroidal anti-inflammatory drugs, and serotonin-norepinephrine reuptake inhibitors (SNRIs).[19] Your medical clinician should work closely with you on which medication or combination of medications may be helpful to try, in an effort to avoid additional side effects and to maximize benefit.[20]

It is important to use caution related to medication prescribed for chronic pain, due to prescription pain medication misuse remaining a significant precipitating and ongoing factor of the national opioid crisis.[23]

Strategies to Try

LISTEN TO YOUR BODY

Building a relationship with our bodies is important for everyone, especially those struggling with chronic pain or illness. Do you know your body's cues, and more importantly, do you honor them? It can be tempting to disregard your body or try to power through, but this will ultimately do you a disservice.

"Parts work" modalities, such as Internal Family Systems Therapy (see page 60), are powerful learning methods to notice and listen to all parts of yourself. By getting to know your body you can "befriend" it, which has been linked to a reduction in pain.[24] You can get to know your parts at home through the books and apps named in the Resources section, or you can pursue "parts work" therapy or coaching.

TAKE ADVANTAGE OF THE FAMILY AND MEDICAL LEAVE ACT

Have an open conversation with your health clinician about potential accommodations through the Family and Medical Leave Act (FMLA) that may enable you to continue engaging in meaningful work. You could ask the clinician about FMLA paperwork that may allow you to have accommodations at work while still protecting your job. This could include working shorter shifts, being able to take breaks after a specific amount of time, or taking time off to attend medical appointments. FMLA may help to protect your position, and thereby your health insurance if you have it through your employer, but it cannot mandate your employer to pay you for time missed at work. Some employers do provide options for paid leave, which may include using your paid-time-off (PTO) allowance.

You may feel reluctant to take FMLA or use other accommodations. We understand that it can be hard to accept help, especially if you know the pain is going to be long-term. We encourage you to check out chapter 10, particularly page 104, to learn more about how setting boundaries (which can include taking FMLA or using other accommodations) can help.

20

CHRONIC PAIN

USE VISUALIZATION AND MEDITATION

Visualization (imagining something good in your mind's eye, such as feeling relaxed and happy) and meditation have long been used by those with chronic pain to bring temporary relief. Research suggests that visualization results in "time shrinkage" (making the duration of the pain seem shorter), or a feeling of distance from the pain even though it still exists.[25] In the words of one study, while visualization cannot actually relieve pain, "some patients created their own internal reality where they could exclude the pain or 'not go into the pain' even though they experienced it."[26]

Similarly, using mindfulness meditation to cope with pain may increase your quality of life and decrease the associated depression and anxiety, even if it does not reduce the pain itself.[27]

The elimination of pain is not the goal of these strategies, but they can make it easier to cope with, which can in turn provide some relief.

ENGAGE IN MANAGEABLE PHYSICAL ACTIVITY

If you have chronic pain, it's likely that you've reduced your physical activity, which can sometimes result in more pain.[28] You can experience pain from both overuse and underuse of muscles. It's important to slowly and incrementally identify a level of activity that works well for you.

Physical activity in general is unlikely to cause harm if you have chronic pain. Even if you worry it will increase your pain further, it is actually likely to help reduce it.[29] If your body allows for it, try to always schedule some kind of physical activity into your daily routine. Despite how difficult this feels when you are in pain, doing so may reduce pain and prevent deterioration in the long run.

ADJUST YOUR EXPECTATIONS OF YOURSELF DAY BY DAY

Spoon Theory was coined in the chronic illness community to explain what it's like to live within a body that is often exhausted and in pain, and to combat the expectations of ableism. Each spoon represents a quantity of energy that gets used up while completing daily tasks, such as getting out of bed or preparing meals. Some days you start with more spoons, and thus can accomplish more things before running out, and other days you have fewer. Everyone's "spoon allotment" is different and it varies day by day.

Activity Pacing is an example of Spoon Theory in action, in which you break down activities into smaller steps (for example, doing the dishes in five-minute chunks) and take breaks in between.

Once the spoons have been used up, they are gone, and cannot come back until the next day. People with chronic pain or illness will use Spoon Theory to measure how much energy they will have available in their day and to make decisions accordingly. If a holiday or outing will eat up most of your daily allotment of spoons, it may be important to get extra help for daily tasks that week.

USE ACTIVE COPING STRATEGIES

Active coping means using strategies to control pain despite your level of pain, while passive coping means you have relinquished the control of your pain to others, like your medical clinician.[30] Active coping could include any of the strategies mentioned in this chapter, such as attending physical therapy appointments, practicing meditation, or talking to loved ones about your spoons.

Your resilience, coping strategies, and self-efficacy (the belief in your ability to meet challenges and achieve goals) can help you experience less daily interference from your pain.[31] If you use passive coping strategies, you are more likely to experience psychological distress and depression, whereas active coping will likely reduce your psychological distress.[32]

Barriers to Feeling Better

NEGATIVE THOUGHTS ABOUT YOUR PAIN

Risk and vulnerability factors such as distress, trauma, fear, and catastrophizing (expecting bad outcomes related to your pain) may increase your risk for and worsen your experience of pain and its disability, burden, or impact.[33] Your thoughts and beliefs about your pain and its intensity can have a powerful impact on how long it persists. Research shows that individuals' beliefs that their back pain would persist was a significant predictor of poor outcome at six months and at five years.[34]

AVOIDANCE RELATED TO YOUR PAIN

For some types of pain, fear of movement or movement-related injury increases the risk of future chronic pain and disability,[35] so you may find yourself avoiding activities that you fear will worsen your pain. However, avoiding use of certain muscles due to such worry may actually result in you experiencing increased pain. At your own pace, strive to find a level of activity that helps you avoid a cycle of avoidance and overuse.

Research tends to see men as the default, assessing "normal" pain reactions based on them, rather than seeing differences in sexes.[36] Women are often not taken as seriously as men when presenting with chronic pain, and their pain is often dismissed as psychological instead of physical.[37]

How to Communicate About Chronic Pain

IF YOU'RE THE ONE WITH CHRONIC PAIN

Consider talking to your loved ones about "Spoon Theory" (see page 202). Talking about your spoons can be a helpful communication shorthand. Share with others the ways in which you hope to be included in activities and discuss accessibility or other accommodations (places to sit, times for rest, scooter availability). It is important to stress your understanding that activities do not need to revolve around you and if attending that event doesn't work out, that you would still like to be invited in the future. Don't be afraid to ask for help but be mindful of other people's limits and boundaries.

IF A LOVED ONE HAS CHRONIC PAIN

You may find that talking about Spoon Theory helps you both. You can discuss how many spoons a planned activity may consume and plan accordingly. Tell your loved ones of plans well in advance and take into consideration any physical barriers in the space, as this can help both of you problem-solve so they can be included. Be mindful that their pain experience can vary from day to day and that just because they were able to complete a task yesterday doesn't mean they will easily be able to do so today. Encourage them to break down tasks into smaller steps and to take frequent breaks. Don't treat your loved one like they are incapable of being active, they just may need to complete the task in a different way. What is important is for them to know they are still included and capable.

You may be tempted to offer unsolicited advice to your loved one, out of a desire to feel helpful. However, they have likely heard this advice many times, and it can be both frustrating and exhausting to be on the receiving end. It can also have the opposite effect of what's intended and they may feel like more of a burden. If there's something important you'd like to communicate about a possible treatment option, ask for permission. You could say something like, "I heard about this promising treatment option, let me know if it'd be helpful to talk about it in the future." Then, if they choose to do so, your loved one can come to you on their own time when they have enough spoons.

IF THE PERSON WITH CHRONIC PAIN IS A CHILD

The same strategies about routine and movement remain true. See if you can make their involvement in daily tasks into a game or activity, such as by assigning points or using a sticker chart. It's also important for your child to feel active in their care. Empower them to notice their body, advocate for its needs, and take age-appropriate responsibility for managing their condition, such as being involved in strategies to remember to take medication or being an active part of conversations with clinicians, especially if it is a condition they will likely need to manage on their own in adulthood.

What Coping with Chronic Pain Can Look Like in Real Life

Tina used to be a dancer. She was always physically fit and able to move her body with ease. A few weeks ago, she started to notice pain in several areas of her body. Being unsure of the cause, she scheduled an appointment with her primary care clinician. At the appointment, she explains that she's found it hard to sleep throughout the night due to her pain, and that it's caused her to shorten her daily walks.

The clinician tells Tina they will check her blood work and encourages her to put warm compresses on the affected areas. They also tell her that she can take non-steroidal anti-inflammatory drugs like ibuprofen or naproxen to help manage the pain.

Tina follows the clinician's instructions, but after another month the pain still feels like an eight out of ten most days. Since her previous lab work was normal, she's referred for a scan and encouraged to consider physical

> **THE RESEARCH SAYS . . .**
>
> **You May Also Experience These Things**
>
> Chronic pain has an association with depression (page 8) and anxiety (page 19).[38] Moreover, having both depression and anxiety further increases your risk of experiencing a number of physical conditions that may then lead to chronic pain.[39]

therapy. She's dismayed when she's told that the scan did not find a cause for her pain.

Tina begins to worry that her pain won't get better. But, having previously been a dancer, she feels like physical therapy may be worthwhile and she starts going to sessions twice a week.

At her next follow-up, Tina tells her primary care clinician that she's noticed some improvements from the physical therapy but is still frustrated that the source of the pain cannot be found. The clinician explains that they will continue to work with her to see if there is an identifiable source of the pain. They encourage her to consider ways in which she can care for herself from a biopsychosocial approach, such as meeting with a pain psychologist and reengaging with her social network, as Tina shared that she had been isolating herself.

Tina finds the therapy sessions helpful in recognizing and reframing her unhelpful thoughts related to her pain. She also starts using the strategy of activity pacing, breaking her daily tasks into smaller steps. She finds that this helps her avoid the cycle of being overactive on days when her pain is manageable and paying for it with increased pain the next day. She also invites some friends over, and finds they are empathetic about her situation and want to know how they can support her.

Tina starts to realize that daily pain may be part of her new normal, but that doesn't mean it gets to have total control of her life.

READING LIST AND OTHER RESOURCES

The Pain Management Workbook: Powerful CBT and Mindfulness Skills to Take Control of Pain and Reclaim Your Life by Rachel Zoffness uses a biopsychosocial approach and scientifically supported interventions rooted in Cognitive Behavioral Therapy, mindfulness, and neuroscience to help you take control of your pain.

When Things Fall Apart: Heart Advice for Difficult Times by Buddhist monk Pema Chödrön describes her experiences accepting painful life circumstances. While it's written primarily about emotional pain, we have found it can be helpful if you are experiencing chronic physical pain that you cannot change.

Books *No Bad Parts* by Richard Schwartz, *The Tender Parts* by Ilyse Kennedy, and *Sacred Medicine* by Lissa Rankin can help you use a "parts work" modality to get to know and listen to what your body is telling you.

This Is Not What I Ordered: Conversations on Chronic Illness, Loss, and Change is a podcast by therapist Lauren Selfridge that explores what it's like to live and cope with chronic illness.

Everything Happens with Kate Bowler is a podcast that takes a candid look at the hardships of life from the perspective of a cancer survivor.

Curable is a paid app that uses the biopsychosocial approach to teach subscribers ways to manage pain.

The app IFS Guide walks people through communicating with their parts, including their body, in order to befriend them.

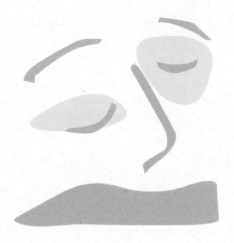

21

SLEEP

A re you tired? Having a bad night of sleep now and then is common, however a lasting pattern over three or more months of difficulty falling, staying, or falling back to sleep after waking in the middle of the night may mean you have insomnia.[1] Sleep is essential to both physical and mental health,[2] and getting *good* sleep can be a challenge.

Chronic difficulty with sleep impacts your ability to function in all areas of your life, as it may negatively impact your mood, ability to think clearly, as well as your heart and brain health, safety while driving, and work-related accidents.[3] Moreover, insomnia increases risk for depression, anxiety, alcohol use disorder, and psychosis.[4] Even children are at risk for issues across all domains of life, including behavior and academic performance, if they do not sleep well.[5] The CDC has declared insufficient sleep a public health epidemic.[6] Sometimes, being aware of the diagnostic criteria can help us take our sleep seriously. The diagnosis of insomnia involves the following.[7]

- Trouble falling asleep, staying asleep, falling back to sleep after waking, or early morning awakening with trouble falling back to sleep, at least three nights per week.

- Sleep difficulties for at least three months.

- Trouble sleeping despite adequate opportunity for sleep.

It is recommended that we get at least seven hours of sleep a night "to support optimal health in adults,"[8] and yet more than a third of adults are estimated to fail to get an optimal amount.[9]

There are many potential factors and diagnoses that may also impede good sleep. Some examples include restless legs syndrome, breathing-related sleep disorders (for example, obstructive sleep apnea), narcolepsy, sleep terrors, sleepwalking, nightmare disorder, and shift work (for example, working at night).[10]

If you are struggling with sleep, it is always advised to speak with a clinician. In tandem with seeking medical guidance, the following sections provide information on recognizing, as well as some considerations for treating, insomnia.

What Professional Help May Look Like

Your schedule may require you to sleep during the day and be awake at night. In the following we describe sleeping at night, but the strategies can be applied to your personal sleep schedule.

COGNITIVE BEHAVIORAL THERAPY FOR INSOMNIA

Cognitive Behavioral Therapy for Insomnia (CBT-I) is the frontline, evidence-based treatment for insomnia.[11] CBT-I is a combination of Cognitive Therapy coupled with behavioral treatments (for example, sleep logs, in which you record the information around your sleep, such as how long it took you to fall asleep and how many times you woke before your alarm went off).[12] Cognitive Therapy seeks to change your negative thoughts and unrealistic expectations of sleep. Common unhelpful thoughts that are identified and addressed in the course of treatment include "I need medication to sleep"; "If I can't sleep I should stay in bed and rest"; and "My life will be ruined if I can't sleep." Such thoughts can create a negative pattern of thinking that may make you feel more stuck in insomnia. It's important to catch and reframe such thoughts, so that you aren't subtly sabotaging your incremental sleep improvements.

MEDICATION

Short courses of medication can supplement CBT or other behavioral therapies, but there is no consensus about how long taking medication will remain effective.[13] While you may benefit from a sleep aid in the short term, if you are able to improve the quality of your sleep using CBT-I and/or at-home techniques you could create lasting change in your sleep patterns. Before starting a sleep aid, please consult your medical clinician.

Strategies to Try

PRACTICE GOOD SLEEP HYGIENE

Practicing sleep hygiene means keeping a regular sleep schedule, having a healthy diet, getting regular daytime exercise, maintaining a quiet sleep environment, and avoiding caffeine, other stimulants, nicotine, alcohol, excessive fluids, or stimulating activities before bedtime.[14]

Sleep hygiene is an important basic step for everyone who sleeps, but it's important to note that it does not have evidence as a solo treatment for chronic insomnia. If you're suffering with insomnia, it should be used in conjunction with stimulus control, which is part of CBT-I, as outlined in the following.

- **Go to bed only when sleepy.** A component of stimulus control is to go to bed only when sleepy. Sleepiness is different from feeling tired; it is when your eyelids feel heavy and it's hard for you to remain awake. You might feel this way, for example, when you start to doze or unintentionally close your eyes while watching TV on the couch.

- **Maintain a regular sleep schedule.** Keep a regular schedule by waking up at the same time each morning, no matter what time you fell asleep or how much sleep you were able to get that night. Figure out a time (such as 7 AM) that it is reasonable for you to wake each day of the week, including on your weekend, and get up at that same time every day. This can feel hard, especially if you're sleep deprived, but we encourage you to try it for a period of time. You may find that a regular sleep schedule, even on weekends, results in better sleep and more energy.

- **Avoid naps.** Avoiding sleep during your routine wake time is important. Although naps can be tempting, especially when you're not getting enough sleep at night, they may be hurting your ability to fall and stay asleep. Your brain may not help you get enough sleep at night if it thinks you can sleep during the day instead. By avoiding naps, you can retrain your brain to understand that the only time you want it to sleep is at night. Try resting without sleeping instead of napping.

- **Use your bed only for sleep and sex.** As much as possible, avoid doing anything aside from sleeping and having sex in bed. You want to teach your brain that bed is where it should be helping you get sleepy. If you do active things, like scroll on your phone or watch TV while in bed, you have likely confused your brain about what you want it to do for you: help you sleep.

- **Get out of bed.** If you're unable to fall asleep or get back to sleep within approximately twenty minutes (don't watch the clock—just feel it out), remove yourself from bed and do a relaxing activity until you feel drowsy, then return to bed. Repeat this as necessary. You want your brain to associate your bed with sleep, so lying in bed awake for more than around twenty minutes is sending it the wrong message. It's often helpful to invest in a slightly boring, but not painfully so, book that you can take to another room and read when you're unable to sleep. However long it takes, sit in soft lighting, in a comfortable chair, and read that slightly boring book until you feel sleepy, and then return to bed.

CREATE A COZY SLEEP ENVIRONMENT

If you do shift work that means you have to sleep during the day, it can be helpful to ensure that the room is dark and cool when you go to sleep. Blackout curtains and/or a sleep mask can be helpful to block out any sunlight. You may also want to find a white noise machine or use earplugs to give another layer of comfort to block out any daytime noise.

KID-FRIENDLY TIP KEEP A WORRY BOX OR WORRY JOURNAL

Try having older children enter their anxieties into a worry box or worry journal before bed. They can draw, write, or cut out magazine photos that represent things they worry about. Before sleep, they can place those things in the box or journal and remind themselves when they are lying awake that their worries are safely out of the way and they will deal with them tomorrow.

ESTABLISH A RELAXING BEDTIME ROUTINE
Having a relaxing bedtime tea or a bedtime stretch routine will help both you and your child wind down without the use of screens.

USE A DREAM CATCHER OR DREAM BOX
A dream catcher or dream box can be helpful for children who have nightmares. Create a story together around how those items help keep them safe from nightmares.

GET GROUNDED
Teach kids the 5-4-3-2-1 method for grounding themselves when they wake up from nightmares. Have them name and describe the following.

- 5 things they can see (a night-light helps with this)
- 4 things they can touch (stuffed animals count!)
- 3 things they can hear (a sound machine with a variety of soothing noises or a familiar audiobook can help)
- 2 things they can smell (like a scented lotion on their nightstand)
- 1 thing they can taste (like a cup of water by the bed)

Barriers to Getting a Good Night's Sleep

NIGHT SHIFT WORK
Working the night shift or doing shift work can make it difficult to get the kind of sleep that is considered optimal. While this can be difficult to change as long as your work shifts remain the same, some of the strategies outlined in this chapter, may still be helpful.

SLEEPING WITH A DISRUPTIVE PARTNER
You may get more restful sleep when sleeping alone. (This includes not getting kicked in the ribs by your kids at night, or having your face stepped on by the cat!) It can be appropriate and healthy to have separate beds or rooms to sleep in if you are disrupted by a partner (or pet). If you think your partner may be interfering with your sleep, consider having a kind and open dialogue with them about sleeping separately. Mutually agreeing to sleep separately doesn't mean there's anything wrong with

you or your relationship. It may actually be a clear investment in each other's health.

HAVING LIMITED HOME SPACE

While stimulus control for sleep tells us to avoid using the bedroom for anything other than sleep and sex, not everyone has enough space to make this a reality. Even if you don't have another room to go to, it's important to get out of the bed or chair where you sleep to avoid lying awake at night. To create a sense of separation, try investing in another chair you can sit in, or moving the chair to a different space when you are reading at night.

How to Communicate About Sleep Difficulties

IF YOU'RE THE ONE EXPERIENCING SLEEP DIFFICULTIES

Speak openly with your loved ones about the strategies you're trying to use to improve your sleep. You could try showing them this chapter or asking them to help you stick to your goals, such as not allowing electronics in bed or sleeping in separate spaces.

Be kind and place the reason for changing behavior on yourself when asking for help. You could say, "I've been struggling with getting good sleep for the last six months. I'm hoping to try out different research-supported strategies to improve my sleep. These changes may help improve my energy during the day when we spend quality time together, and they may include us sleeping apart or my needing to get out of bed at night. I will be as quiet as possible when doing this. Can I ask for your support in this?"

IF A LOVED ONE IS EXPERIENCING SLEEP DIFFICULTIES

Ask how you can support their goals and be open to changing some of your behavior to help them. You could say, "What ideas do you have about how I can best support you in getting good rest at night?"

IF THE PERSON EXPERIENCING SLEEP DIFFICULTIES IS A CHILD

Keep in mind that parent-child sleep is considered bidirectional, meaning that each of your sleep habits impact the other person.[15] Any parent who has ever had their sleep interrupted by a toddler or child with a nightmare can tell you that. The good news is that when you repair your sleep, you may be helping your child sleep better, too.

Gently explore with your child what they feel is interfering with their sleep and, without dismissing their concerns, try to increase their comfort with staying in their own bed.

Sleep routines are important for children. Managing children's anxiety at bedtime is an important part of getting good sleep, and although it can be hard to accept, overuse of screen time leads to sleep disruptions for children.[16]

What Coping with Insomnia Can Look Like in Real Life

Zack hasn't been a "good sleeper" for what feels like his entire adult life. The older he's gotten, the worse his sleep has gotten. He figures it's part of being a grown-up, and that after the days of summer vacation in high school, no one gets good sleep anymore. Most nights he lies awake scrolling on his phone for hours. He has trouble falling and staying asleep at night. He gets a total of four hours of sleep a night, at most. He watches TV in bed trying to fall asleep and will lie in bed awake for hours if he wakes in the middle of the night and can't fall back to sleep.

It isn't until a discussion with a close friend that he starts thinking that maybe not everyone is up half the night. He looks up "insomnia" and finds that there is a treatment available called CBT-I. The next month, he's sitting across from a psychologist who confirms that he does in fact have a diagnosable case of insomnia, and that, thankfully, treatment is available.

Using the strategies discussed in therapy, Zack avoids using electronic devices while in bed. He also avoids exercise, caffeine, and alcohol in the three hours prior to bedtime. At first he misses that after-dinner espresso, but the results are worth it. He learns to go to bed only when sleepy, meaning when his eyelids feel heavy and difficult to keep open, and to get out of bed if unable to fall asleep or get back to sleep within 20 minutes. He also starts to get up at the same time each day regardless of how much sleep he got the night before, being mindful of safety in his functioning the rest of that day. This means having to let go of his dream of repeating those lazy high school days of summer vacation. Instead of feeling discouraged by thoughts such as *My sleep will never get better*, he reframes the thought to *My sleep isn't where I want it to be yet, but that doesn't mean it will never get better*. After consistently practicing these strategies, Zack starts to notice an improvement in his quantity and quality of sleep.

READING LIST AND OTHER RESOURCES

Why We Sleep is a popular book about the science of sleep written by Matthew Walker. This book can help you understand why your brain and body need sleep, and how to harness its power to your advantage.

Rest Is Resistance: A Manifesto by Tricia Hersey is a wonderful book that examines lack of sleep as a part of capitalism and white supremacy and invites us to view rest as a way to heal our cultural trauma.

The Nap Ministry's Rest Deck is Tricia Hersey's illustrated deck of cards—invitations to rest and sleep. The Nap Ministry (thenapministry.com) provides many additional resources to encourage sleep.

The website of the American Academy of Sleep Medicine (sleepeducation.org/healthy-sleep) provides instruction about what healthy sleep looks like across the lifespan, as well as other resources. Not everything is one-size-fits-all, but this may give you a framework to work from.

The National Sleep Foundation's website provides a list of CBT-I clinicians. If you cannot afford CBT-I therapy, the app CBT-i Coach is aimed at helping you use the evidence-based strategies of CBT for Insomnia.

Sleep stories are gentle bedtime stories told in a soothing tone that often help people drift off to sleep. They are available for both children and adults. If you are interested in finding some sleep stories that work for you, there are many available online.

5

GETTING SUPPORT

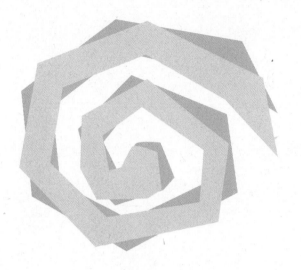

2 2

NAVIGATING THE MENTAL HEALTH SYSTEM

I f you feel overwhelmed every time you try to seek mental health treatment for yourself or a loved one, you are not alone. Navigating the options, jargon, and pitfalls of the United States's mental health system can be difficult even for mental health professionals. As therapists, we often receive outreach from people who are just trying to understand what they should do first. Should they call their insurance? Should they go to a local emergency room seeking treatment? What happens if they don't like their therapist or if their therapist does something wrong? In this chapter, we aim to provide you with a framework to understand the US mental health system and some tools to help you along the way.

GETTING SUPPORT

A Quick Guide to Therapy Terminology

Therapy-related mental health terminology can be confusing. Below, we define some common therapy terms you may encounter.

The terms **"client"** and **"patient"** are often used interchangeably in the mental health system. In this chapter, we use "client" to mean a person being seen in an outpatient or office setting, and a "patient" to mean someone seen in an inpatient or hospital setting, although this is not always how these terms are used.

Outpatient therapy is what you likely think of as "therapy." It's usually conducted once or twice a week with the same therapist each time, for a duration of several months to years. The purpose of outpatient therapy is to work on specific life goals or problems, such as the topics we've discussed in this book. Outpatient therapy is generally the lowest level of care in terms of intensity.

Intensive therapy happens in a traditional outpatient setting, but for several full days in a row. Intensive therapy is evidence based for certain diagnoses, such as Post-Traumatic Stress Disorder, and requires that you are stable enough to engage in intense weeklong therapy. Intensive therapy is not a replacement for intensive outpatient (IOP), partial, or inpatient treatment.

An **intensive outpatient program (IOP)** is one level of care below a partial hospitalization program. Every IOP is different, but they usually take place a few times a week and feature a combination of group and individual therapy and medication management. IOPs are often specialized, such as Dialectical Behavioral Therapy IOP, Eye Movement Desensitization and Reprocessing IOP, or drug and alcohol recovery IOP. An IOP can be a good choice if you know you need specialized support but do not need the security of a hospital.

Partial hospitalization is one level of care below inpatient hospitalization. Partial hospitalization programs are usually daily, featuring a combination of group and individual therapy plus medication management. You will sleep at home and attend a partial program throughout the day. You may attend a partial hospitalization program when you are being transitioned from an inpatient program, so you can gradually return to your usual life. Other times, you may attend a partial hospitalization in an effort not to be admitted to the hospital.

Receiving **inpatient therapy or inpatient services** means that you are currently admitted to a hospital setting, usually a psychiatric or behavioral health hospital, while you are receiving mental health treatment. Inpatient therapy is considered the highest level of care for when you need more support than outpatient therapy can provide, if you are actively harming yourself, or if you are a threat to someone else's safety.

You may enter an inpatient setting at your own free will because you feel too overwhelmed to stay at home. However, you also may be **"involuntarily committed,"** meaning that someone else, such as a hospital social worker or police officer, made the decision that you needed inpatient-level care for safety reasons. Once you have been involuntarily committed, you usually need to stay a certain length of time, such as seventy-two hours, and demonstrate that you can keep yourself and others safe, before being discharged. Please see our Resources section for information about what to do if this has happened to you unfairly.

Drug and alcohol treatment is its own specialized field, with its own tiered system. If you enter drug and alcohol treatment while you are still using, you typically need to detox first, in order to safely manage withdrawal symptoms. Detox is closely managed by medical staff and the length of time varies for every situation, but it can take up to several weeks. After you complete the detox, you may transition to a rehabilitation program, or you may participate in outpatient therapy or a twelve-step recovery group such as Alcoholics Anonymous or Narcotics Anonymous. The team overseeing your treatment would make recommendations for your specific placement. While in drug and alcohol recovery, you may graduate to a recovery house or sober living house for ongoing community support, or become sponsored and then eventually sponsor others in a twelve-step group.

Finding the Right Treatment for You

If you find yourself or a loved one in need of any of these mental health treatments, start by asking trusted friends or family if they have recommendations. The best places to go will be different from one community to the next. Like medical treatment, quality mental health treatment in any setting is dependent on the clinicians who are providing the service.

It will be important to check your insurance coverage as well. This can often be found through your insurance online portal or by calling the number on the back of your insurance card (for more, check out chapter 26).

KID-FRIENDLY TIP As with a medical diagnosis, there are some highly complicated cases that can require outside support to connect to the right clinicians and treatment centers. If you have a child who is navigating a complicated mental health diagnosis, a therapeutic educational consultant can help.

Therapeutic educational consultants advocate for your child, assist with managing placements in the child mental health system, and can help you navigate the impact of a mental health placement on the child's school setting. You can find them at the National Association of Therapeutic Schools and Programs or by searching online.

For adults, a great resource to find a peer specialist is the National Alliance on Mental Illness. Peer specialists have experienced their own mental health situations and are there to help you through yours.

Case managers may also be available, often through community mental health agencies, to help you navigate the health care system.

Barriers to Finding Treatment

LACKING THE ENERGY, MOTIVATION, OR CLARITY TO SEEK HELP

One of the most difficult parts of navigating a mental health diagnosis is how it impacts your functioning. If you are depressed, anxious, experiencing insomnia, Post-Traumatic Stress Disorder symptoms, or any number of the other diagnoses we have discussed in this book, it may feel nearly impossible to have the energy or clarity to connect with the right mental health resources. If this is you, please reach out to someone like a trusted friend or family member for help connecting with the treatment option that is best for you.

However, we know many people experiencing mental health concerns are often isolated. If you don't have close friends or family members you can turn to, a peer specialist or case manager could help. Community mental health resources may also be available to you; see chapter 24. If you are part of a faith community, this may also give you access to other resources for connecting you with the mental health care you need.

LONG WAIT TIMES

Since the COVID-19 pandemic began, the already overwhelmed mental health system has gotten even more difficult to navigate. We've heard many stories of people going to their local emergency room to connect with mental health care, only to wait for days to be seen.

A local emergency room is a good place to go if your mental health situation is a true emergency, meaning that you or someone else will be hurt if you don't go. In that case, at least you or the other person will be kept safe while you wait. If what you are experiencing is not an emergency, it may be best to connect with your community mental health resource instead.

If you're on a waiting list for therapy services and it is not an emergency, we hope that the coping skills and resources in this book will help you as you wait.

EXPERIENCING SUBPAR CARE

The quality of care at any of the levels of mental health treatment can vary greatly depending on the skill, compassion, and ethics of the staff. You can always ask for a new treatment clinician if the one you are assigned is not a good fit for you.

If you've been treated unethically by a mental health clinician, you have every right to report them. If they are licensed, you can report them to their licensing board. If not, you can report them to the organization they work for.

In this context, reporting a clinician is considered a serious matter that may result in the person's license being revoked, so it should be used for serious concerns. It may involve you releasing your records and participating in the investigation. If you have a complaint about a less serious concern such as scheduling, you can explain it to the agency or organization you are receiving treatment from without needing to make a formal report.

STIGMA AND SHAME

Worries about how others may perceive you could result in you avoiding reaching out for treatment. In particular, the cultural or gendered beliefs that mental illness equates to a weakness of character, or that it is taboo to talk about, have negative outcomes for the people who often need treatment the most. It may be helpful to speak with a trusted loved one or to seek online treatment from the comfort of your home. Once you are connected to professional support, you can make reducing your feelings of shame one of your treatment goals, if you'd like.

How to Communicate While Navigating the Mental Health System

IF YOU'RE THE ONE NAVIGATING THE MENTAL HEALTH SYSTEM

It can feel vulnerable to communicate with anyone, whether a professional or a friend, about your mental health. Sometimes it's hard to even find the words to express how you are feeling. You can try writing down your experiences to take to your first appointment with a mental health clinician or to share with a loved one as a way to communicate how you've been feeling. You may want to focus on the daily-life impact your mental health is having, and what you hope will change by reaching out. Some people find that putting their words in an email or text message makes it a bit easier than talking face-to-face.

If you have someone you trust enough, see if they can go with you to your initial appointment. Having someone you can be honest in front of with you can help you stay calm and remember all of the important things to share.

IF A LOVED ONE IS NAVIGATING THE MENTAL HEALTH SYSTEM

Sharing one's mental health is vulnerable, so please be patient and gentle with your loved one. Try not to ask why they haven't done something differently yet, or why they are acting a certain way; trust that they are doing the best they can.

The choices about what kind of mental health professional to see and in what kind of setting are highly personal. And the process often takes much longer than expected. If you want to offer support in this process, consider practical support, such as attending the initial appointment if they would like, or driving them to the appointment and going out for coffee afterward.

Try to connect with other parents or caregivers who have had children go through similar things. It is painful to watch your child struggle with their mental health and support can mean everything. Plus, other parents or caregivers can offer you their best tips about the facilities, therapists, and other supports they've found in your community. Many parents find it helpful to join social media groups for parents of children with specific mental health diagnoses.

What Finding Treatment Can Look Like in Real Life

Chris has had some depression and anxiety off and on throughout their life, but never thought it was a big enough deal to seek help. However, after a big life stressor, they find that they can't manage their feelings the way they used to. It's hard to get out of bed in the morning, and they find themself having panic attacks when doing things they used to do easily, like driving.

Chris decides they need a therapist, so they do an online search and send emails to a few who look good. Weeks go by, and they don't hear anything back. They start to feel even more panicky, worrying that they will never get help, and this thought makes them feel worse than ever before.

After reading this book, Chris decides to see if their local community mental health center has walk-in hours. It does, so they rearrange their work schedule one day and go. After waiting for a couple of hours, they see an intake worker who asks questions about how they've been feeling. She lets Chris know that they qualify to see a therapist and a psychiatrist for treatment, and connects them with a caseworker to help them with the paperwork. She lets them know it will be about a month before their first appointment, but she gives them some reading material to help in the meantime.

Knowing they have the appointment coming up makes Chris feel better, and they are able to relax and sleep well for the first time in what feels like months. By the time their appointment date comes, they almost feel so much better they don't go, but they remember how bad they felt before and so they keep their appointment. They're glad they do, because when they meet with the therapist, the therapist explains the symptoms of panic Chris has been experiencing. Plus, their caseworker helps them figure out some complicated paperwork they've been putting off. Understanding themself makes

Chris feel even better, and when they meet with the psychiatrist and they explain that a selective serotonin reuptake inhibitor could help them continue to improve, they feel like they're on track to getting their old life back.

READING LIST AND OTHER RESOURCES

You Are Not Alone: The NAMI Guide to Navigating Mental Health—With Advice from Experts and Wisdom from Real People and Families by Ken Duckworth, MD. This book provides a wealth of knowledge about the mental health system and incorporates many lived experiences, both from the perspectives of those experiencing the struggles as well as their loved ones.

If you have been unfairly involuntarily committed, the organization Project Lets is a texting-based resource for people experiencing urgent issues related to involuntary psychiatric hospitalization. Text them at 401-400-2905 if you have urgent need. They also offer online support groups for people who have experienced harm at the hands of the psychiatric system. Find out more on their website: projectlets.org.

The wait to connect with mental health treatment can be a long and frustrating. While apps are not a replacement for professional treatment, the following list includes some that can be helpful while you wait. (Please note that since the world of apps is constantly changing, some of these may no longer be free or relevant when you read this.)

MindShift helps you use Cognitive Behavioral Therapy tools such as reframing your thoughts.

What's Up uses skills from Cognitive Behavioral Therapy and Acceptance and Commitment Therapy.

PTSD Coach is designed by Veterans Affairs. It has tools such as breathing and mindfulness exercises to help you manage your PTSD symptoms.

The Insight Timer guides you through meditations for calming and sleep.

The Shine App is designed specifically to support the mental health experiences of people of color.

Better Stop Suicide aims to bring calm if you are experiencing suicidal ideation. It is not meant to be a replacement for emergency mental health care.

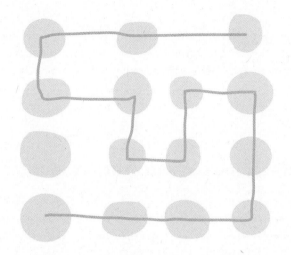

23

NAVIGATING A MENTAL HEALTH CRISIS

N o one ever wants to experience a mental health crisis. A mental health crisis is a situation in which your mental health–related behaviors put you at risk of harming yourself or others, or it prevents you from being able to care for yourself and function. It interrupts the normal flow of life, throwing it into complete upheaval.[1]

If you are experiencing a mental health crisis, you may notice the following.

- You withdraw from your friends and favorite activities.

- Your emotions, especially sadness, irritability, hopelessness, and even happiness, feel more extreme than usual, and you cannot manage them.

- You feel unusually forgetful, tired, unmotivated, or paranoid.

- You have a poor appetite, aren't sleeping, and/or aren't taking care of your basic hygiene.

- You're thinking, saying, or doing things that seem bizarre to you.

- You feel as if you are not connected to or a part of reality.

- You're using substances more than usual or in an unsafe way.

- You're thinking about harming or killing yourself.[2]

While many people live with mental illnesses their whole lives without experiencing a crisis, you might experience a mental health crisis because of circumstances such as increased life stress, experiencing a trauma, or using or stopping use of a substance. If you've experienced a mental health crisis or have a loved one you're worried about, please read on for some important considerations.

What Professional Help May Look Like

Evidence-based treatment is important during mental health emergencies. All mental health treatment should be trauma-informed, meaning it centers on your individual choices and personhood and provides options whenever possible. There are some specific modalities that have been proven to be effective when a person is experiencing increased mental health symptoms, such as suicidal ideation. The Collaborative Assessment and Management of Suicidality (CAMS) approach, which helps you both openly discuss your reasons for dying and identify your reasons for living, has been shown to decrease hopelessness in some populations.[3] Therapy models such as Cognitive Behavioral Therapy and Dialectical Behavioral Therapy can assist you in changing your thoughts and behaviors around suicidality. Selective serotonin reuptake inhibitors (SSRIs) have shown to be effective if you are experiencing suicidal ideation at any age, and ketamine-assisted therapy may be helpful if you have treatment-resistant depression.[7]

How to Manage a Mental Health Crisis

The best thing you can do to manage a mental health crisis is to have a realistic crisis plan in place before one happens. Conventional wisdom says that when you're experiencing a mental health crisis, your first step should be to call 911 or 988 (the National Suicide and Crisis Lifeline). While these options work for some, they don't feel safe to everyone, particularly if you have traumatic experiences or concerns related to police or involuntary hospitalization.

Some areas of the country have mobile crisis teams, which may include social workers, that can be deployed to your home to assess your needs during a mental health emergency. These mobile crisis programs are designed to help you avoid inpatient psychiatric hospitalizations whenever possible. You may prefer to receive a mobile crisis assessment instead of interacting with law enforcement.

There are also numerous "warm lines," or peer support hotlines, which you can call to receive support from people who have been through experiences similar to yours. You may find this feels more supportive than speaking to a professional. Warm lines will often suggest reaching out to a professional if they think you could benefit from additional support.

Some apps allow you to input a personalized crisis plan so that if you feel too overwhelmed by depression or anxiety in the moment, you can go to your app and easily access your resources. Consider putting your local warm line number in the app, as well as those of online support groups or peer-run groups, and any other supports you want to use during a crisis. Check out the Resources section of this chapter for some suggestions of apps and groups. Make sure to fill in your crisis plan in these apps when you are not in a crisis, so that you are mentally able to access all potential ideas and resources.

You can also create your own "portable treatment record," which details your prior mental health history, your treatment history, your medications, and your preferences for treatment. The National Alliance on Mental Illness provides a free outline, or you can input this information into an app. By doing so, your mental health history and treatment wishes will be available to you even if you can't remember them in the middle of a crisis.

If you have a friend or family member who you trust, make them a part of your crisis plan. On a good day, talk to them about your preferences when it comes to dealing with a mental health emergency. Consider listing your preferences in order of what you feel most to least comfortable with, so that they know what to try first. For example, you may prefer to start with a mobile crisis team or by calling your primary therapist or psychiatrist, and to call 911 as a last resort. Having a trusted person who can walk you through the steps when you feel overwhelmed or depressed can help. If you know that when you enter a dark place it's too hard to reach out with words, consider having a "crisis emoji." Sending this emoji to a friend will instantly let them know you need help.

The National Suicide and Crisis Lifeline (988) is not a perfect resource, but it is continuously listening to feedback and working to become a better option for people in crisis, including by reviewing all calls that end up being referred to law enforcement, and training operators on the alternatives.[8] The 988 lifeline also has services available for the deaf and hard of hearing. When you call 988, your call will be routed to a local crisis response agency who will be aware of the mental health resources in your area. A trained crisis counselor will ask you questions about your mental health symptoms and assess what level of care you would benefit from. If needed, they will make a recommendation for next steps.

When accessing any of these resources, please keep in mind that licensed mental health professionals have a legal requirement to take steps if they believe you are in imminent danger because of suicidal or homicidal intentions. These steps are meant to take your exact needs into consideration, including working with you in outpatient therapy as long as you don't have a plan to carry out your suicidal or homicidal thoughts. However, some people report that the next steps involved being involuntarily committed to an inpatient program when they were not a danger to themselves or others, while others report that they needed and wanted to be admitted to an inpatient setting and were told there was not enough room. While mental health professionals are required to undergo regular training to ensure quality of care, particularly when it comes to treating those presenting with suicidal thoughts, the quality and competence of this care varies widely depending on the professional.

When you are speaking to a mental health clinician, whether they're your regular therapist or someone on a hotline, ask them about the policies that govern them when it comes to next steps around suicidal or homicidal intention. Ask if they consider suicidal thoughts without a follow-up plan to be a threat, or if they are willing to work with you as long as you decide not to carry out a plan. Ask what they would do if you did have a plan to kill yourself. Knowing your options ahead of time will empower you when you are experiencing a mental health crisis.

Barriers to Finding Help During a Crisis

SYSTEMIC OBSTACLES

Systemic change is necessary before everyone will feel safe accessing treatment during a mental health crisis. Much needs to be done in order to provide trauma-informed and equitable treatment for all people, especially populations that have been shown to be particularly vulnerable to mistreatment, which includes those with mental illness, neurodivergent people, people of color, and people who identify as LBGTQ+.[9] This needs to include extensive training in crisis management, including simulations, for law enforcement and others who come into contact with people in mental health crises, as well as a national increase in mobile crisis response teams.[10]

PAST EXPERIENCES

Past trauma at the hands of the mental health system can be a serious barrier to you reaching out if you need help. The American mental health system is understaffed and overrun, with extensive waiting lists. Witnessing our clients face the challenge of being unable to find appropriate support is a big component in what drove us to write this book.

The mental health system's reliance upon policing for enforcement during mental health crises has created further barriers and trauma. Specific traumatic experiences, such as being hospitalized against your will or having a violent encounter with law enforcement, may stop you from reaching out for mental health support when you experience a crisis. Since those with mental illness are four times more likely to be shot during a police interaction than other individuals, this hesitation is an understandable survival strategy.[11] Remember that there are options available other than calling 911, such as accessing a mobile crisis program if one is available in your area.

STIGMA AND SHAME

Stigma and shame around mental health emergencies may cause you to avoid seeking appropriate treatment, and it especially abounds in some ethnic and religious cultures, as well as among men. This is especially concerning as these groups often experience more incidents of depression and suicidality, while simultaneously having the least access to treatment.[12]

The long-standing tradition rooted in capitalism, ableism, and racism of our mental health system to quickly silence, incarcerate, or institutionalize people experiencing a mental health crisis remains some of the biggest barriers to equitable, successful mental health treatment. Historically, this discrimination, including criminal justice action instead of mental health support, has impacted minorities the most.[13]

There is still much work to be done, but in 2023 the World Health Organization and United Nations jointly issued a statement suggesting new mental health treatment guidelines.[14] Acknowledging that previous mental health legislation has facilitated discrimination and other harmful practices, the statement advocates for person-centered and community-based services; eradicating stigma, discrimination, and coercion; promoting community inclusion and participation; developing accountability measures; and listening to those with lived experiences, including that of intergenerational trauma. The document also makes the case for the socioeconomic benefits of appropriate mental health treatment.[15]

THE RESEARCH SAYS . . .

You May Also Experience These Things

There is a strong link between mental health crises and substance abuse (page 188).[16] If you're finding yourself experiencing symptoms of a mental health crisis, consider whether you've recently taken any substances that could have caused it. Even some prescription medication can have the unintentional effect of causing a mental health crisis. Make sure to tell any treatment clinicians about the substance you took so they can provide safe and effective care.

How to Communicate About a Mental Health Crisis

IF YOU'RE THE ONE EXPERIENCING A MENTAL HEALTH CRISIS

If at all possible, communicate with your support network before you are actually experiencing a mental health crisis. Share with them what your warning signs look like when you are sliding toward a mental health crisis (for example, not getting out of bed to go to work or school, isolating yourself, not eating regular meals), and coping options that work for you, such as taking a walk with a friend, getting help with daily chores, or increasing the frequency of your therapy visits. Also let them know your preferred mental health crisis plan, including hotlines/warm lines, what your local mobile crisis or online support options are, and, if your plan includes potential inpatient treatment, the facilities you're willing to consider.

IF A LOVED ONE IS EXPERIENCING A MENTAL HEALTH CRISIS

Mental health emergencies are serious matters. While it may appear from the outside that your loved one is able to function as usual and meet their basic needs, chances are that they are experiencing debilitating depression, anxiety, or other symptoms that make it necessary for them to have outside support. If you are available, offer to connect them to services like increased therapy visits or a peer-run group or hotline, and even make the initial phone calls for them if you can. So that you do not burn out, this should be a short-term solution that is used just until your loved one is able to manage these things for themselves, or is connected to a professional who can help, such as a case manager. If you feel you can be available for your loved one in this short-term way, make sure you're still putting your own mental health care needs first. You can set any boundaries or practice any self-care you need. As the analogy goes, you have to put on your own oxygen mask before you help others.

You may feel concerned that talking about your loved one's mental health emergency may make it worse, but you should know that research shows asking a person if they are feeling suicidal does not cause a person to have suicidal thoughts.[17] It is safe to ask direct questions to a person having a mental health emergency, including about how they're doing or feeling. However, if your loved one sets a boundary and says they need space from those questions, it's important to listen to them.

IF THE PERSON EXPERIENCING A MENTAL HEALTH CRISIS IS A CHILD

Our hearts go out to you. Please take care of yourself as your child goes through this hard time. We know it can feel nearly impossible to find time or energy for self-care when your child is going through a crisis, but please find support when you can. Exchange responsibility with other caregivers when possible, focus on having adequate sleep, nutrition, and hygiene, and ask for help with tasks that can be delegated. Your child's mental health is a marathon, not a sprint, and you need to be well resourced for the journey.

When speaking with a child or adolescent, be mindful not to invalidate their feelings and experiences. Approach them with curious and open "we" language, asking gentle questions, such as "How can we make this better?" Children may not have the right language to express their feelings, so be careful not to invalidate their responses, even if what they are saying is not immediately clear to you.

What a Mental Health Crisis Can Look Like in Real Life

Susan has struggled with depression and anxiety for as long as she can remember. She's been in and out of therapy for years now, but it feels hard to practice what she's learned. Her medication is helpful, but when she's having a bad streak, she honestly can't remember to take it.

Almost no one knows how bad it gets sometimes—that she won't leave her bed or eat for days, because she feels so hopeless and lethargic. She feels like a failure. She finds herself thinking *What's wrong with me?*

One day, her sister stops by and sees what a mess her place is. Susan tells her sister that she hasn't been eating and that she doesn't even care if she dies. Her sister says she's going to call someone for help, and Susan immediately begins to panic.

In high school Susan was admitted to a "psych hospital," and it was one of the worst experiences of her life. She was put in an unfamiliar environment with total strangers during an incredibly vulnerable time. Her sister sees her distress, and she calls a mobile crisis team instead. It takes a few hours, but Susan's sister waits with her until the crisis team arrives. When they do, it's two social workers who ask Susan questions about her mental health history and how she's functioning these days.

She's tempted to lie, but her sister is there, so she tells the truth. The social workers explain that since she isn't actively suicidal, Susan can stay at her apartment, but that they'd like her to go to a partial program, where each day she'll have group therapy and a chance to meet with a therapist and psychiatrist.

Susan starts the program the next day. She learns tons of new coping strategies from the group, but she feels pretty hopeless about having the energy to try them.

Then she meets with the psychiatrist, and they explain that they can prescribe an injectable antidepressant so she doesn't have to remember to take it every day. After she regularly has the antidepressant in her system, Susan feels like she can try the coping strategies from the group. She also gets connected with a peer specialist that she can call when she's having a dark day. It feels good to have people in her world who really understand.

READING LIST AND OTHER RESOURCES

The Treatment Advocacy Center (treatmentadvocacycenter.org) provides state-by-state information about laws and policies that govern mental health treatment and grades states on how well they handle mental health concerns.

The National Alliance on Mental Illness (NAMI) has an online resource directory of "warm lines" by geographic area on their website. To find it, you can type "NAMI warm lines" into a search engine, or go to nami.org/help.

Thrive Lifeline is a text-based hotline that does not refer to law enforcement. You can text "Thrive" to 1-313-662-8209 to have a text conversation with them at any time.

BlackLine is a crisis hotline staffed by and geared toward Black, Brown, Indigenous, and individuals who identify as LGBTQ+. Their number is 800-604-5841.

Trans Lifeline is a hotline for trans or questioning people in crisis, with services in English and Spanish. Their number is 877-565-8860.

The Wildflower Alliance (wildfloweralliance.org) is an online resource that hosts peer-run support groups for a wide variety of crisis-related topics.

Project LETS is a text-based resource if you are experiencing urgent issues related to involuntary psychiatric hospitalization. Text them at 401-400-2905 if you have an urgent need. If you do not have access to your phone, you can fill out an online intake form at projectlets.org in their Resources section under Crisis Support. If you do not have access to the internet, you can ask a friend or family member to contact them on your behalf.

SAMHSA's Suicide Safe and the Virtual Hope Box are two apps that you can use to create a virtual crisis plan as referenced in the How to Manage a Mental Health Crisis section on page 228.

24

FINDING A MENTAL HEALTH PROFESSIONAL

F inding the right mental health professional is no easy task. Having a positive relationship with your mental health clinician, sometimes called the "therapeutic alliance," is a critical factor in determining whether or not treatment will be successful.[1] In fact, a great deal of therapy's success is determined by the relationship between the client and therapist.[2] Even more important to your treatment outcomes than the kind of modality the mental health professional uses (such as CBT or EMDR), is whether you feel that you can trust them, and that they show warmth and empathy toward you.[3]

Mental health professionals are trained to treat clients with unconditional positive regard, which is considered one of the central tenets of effective treatment.[4] However, in our therapy practices we hear from people who have had the opposite experience. Some have been judged or shamed by their therapist. Others have been at the receiving end of poor boundaries, ethical violations, and even sexual advances. We've heard more times than we care to admit about clinicians falling asleep in session or taking over the session with their own tales of woe.

In this chapter, we hope to help you navigate the complicated world of finding a mental health professional who is a good fit for you.

What To Expect from a Mental Health Professional

There are numerous factors to consider when you are trying to find the right therapist for you.

PRESENTATION AND PERSONALITY

Everyone is different when it comes to who they feel safe with, and who they can trust with their most vulnerable thoughts and feelings. You may love a therapist with tattoos and piercings who makes you feel like your life choices won't be judged. Alternatively, you may want a gentle, maternal figure, or prefer someone who is direct. Even details such as gender identity, age, religious and political affiliations, and what the therapist's office looks like are important factors in whether you immediately feel connected. However, we want to remind you to not judge a book by its cover. If you are having a tough time finding a therapist you connect with, you may benefit from seeing someone outside of your typical preferences. Maybe they'll be who you've been looking for all along!

TRAINING AND EXPERTISE

While the therapeutic relationship is a crucial predictor of therapy success, it's still true that for the most successful outcome you'll want to see a therapist who has training and expertise in the concern that is bringing you to therapy. Just like you wouldn't go to a dentist if you had a problem with your heart, it's usually best to go to the kind of therapist who specializes in your specific concern. Thankfully, there are certifications in nearly every mental health concern you can think of, from PTSD to eating disorders to Substance Use Disorder.

If you're looking for a therapist for a child, it's best to seek out therapists who specialize in working with children. Within the child therapist specialty, there are therapists who work best with younger children, and others who can help teens.

PROFESSIONALISM AND ETHICS

We wish we didn't have to include this, but we've heard enough therapy horror stories to know we must. When you're seeing a therapist, you are seeing a professional who should be held to certain standards. You have the right to see a therapist who respects your time by not coming to the session late or ending it early. You have the right to see a therapist who makes the entire session *your* time, focusing on you and your needs, not their own needs or agenda.

Your therapist should never have a dual relationship with you, such as asking for your help with a project, to pay for a service unrelated to therapy, or to be your friend or sexual partner. While some therapists use stories or information about themselves to further the therapy goals, the point should always be to help you along, not to focus on themselves. In fact, the ethical consideration therapists are always supposed to consider is whether their help is in *your* best interest. Your therapist should be alert, calm, and focused on you throughout your sessions. While what this looks like can vary greatly from therapist to therapist, and it's a beautiful thing to have therapists with all personalities and styles, you should always feel safe and heard in your sessions.

Your therapist should agree on goals with you from the beginning of the therapeutic relationship, and check in with you about these goals regularly. Your therapist should ideally ask you for feedback about how the therapy is going, but at the very least be open and responsive to the feedback you offer. If something isn't going well in therapy, bring it up with them. We know it's hard to do, but it's worth it to keep an open dialogue about any concerns you may have.

Therapists are people, too, and have bad days just like everyone else. Sometimes a therapist might run late, or appear distracted, or forget something you told them before. When mistakes happen, the therapist should own it and apologize, never minimize it or blame it on you. By repairing attachment ruptures in the therapeutic relationship, the therapist can give you a model and practice for your other relationships.

Most therapists will have a brief phone or telehealth chat with clients who want to learn more about working with them. This conversation is not therapy, it's a "good fit" consultation to determine if you think you'd like to move forward. It's also an opportunity for the therapist to tell you if they don't think they'd be the right fit for you. To prepare for the call, try to be as specific as you can about the kind of therapist you are looking for. Also, ask about payment and insurance, how long the therapist's sessions typically last, and for an estimate of how many times you'll plan to meet initially.

The initial appointment with a therapist is usually called an intake appointment. At the intake, you can usually expect to provide a history of your mental health, medical health, and the current issue you are seeking therapy for, as well as information about your family, daily functioning, and what goals you'd like to achieve from therapy.

A Quick Guide to Different Types of Mental Health Professionals

The therapy world can feel overwhelming when you're trying to figure out what kind of therapist is best for you. Even the terminology itself can be confusing! Below we review common types of mental health professionals you may encounter in the US. (Note that depending on your state's requirements and how long ago the professional earned their degree, some professionals may have different qualifications than those listed here.)

A **psychiatrist** has an advanced medical degree (MD or a DO) and can diagnose and prescribe medications for mental health concerns. Psychiatrists will meet with you, often monthly, to discuss your medication needs.

A **psychiatric nurse practitioner** has a different degree (such as a CRNP) than a psychiatrist, but they can often prescribe psychiatric medication in much the same way.

A **psychologist** has a doctorate with a specialized focus on psychology (PsyD, PhD, EdD) and provides both therapy and assessments. Assessments vary in their purpose, for example, a custody evaluation during a divorce or to diagnose ADHD, but they will likely contain a thorough interview and a battery of tests. Psychologists specialize in different areas as they obtain their degree. Some examples include counseling psychology and clinical psychology.

A **licensed clinical social worker** has a graduate degree (LSW or LCSW) that allows them to consider the sociological issues that you face. For example, they may be uniquely qualified to help you process your mental health in the context of your race, or to help you advocate for your needs within systems such as the criminal justice system.

A **licensed therapist** (LPC) has obtained a minimum of a master's degree in psychology or a related field, has met the standards of their state's licensing board, and can provide therapy sessions. Licensed therapists may have extra certifications in any number of specialties.

A **pre-licensed clinician** is undergoing the process for licensure. Because this is a multi-year process, the person is supervised by a licensed therapist who usually sees the same kinds of clients, although the pre-licensed clinician cannot become certified in some therapy modalities until they are fully licensed.

A **practicum student/therapy intern/extern** is a graduate student in a master's or doctoral program who is practicing therapy under the supervision of a licensed clinician. Trainees are usually practicum students or interns for two to five years, depending on their program. After that training, they may choose to become a pre-licensed clinician and then eventually a licensed clinician.

A **mental health clinician** is an umbrella term for someone who practices therapy with clients, not someone who is not solely focused on research. Some therapists prefer the term "clinician." Moreover, "provider" is a term insurance companies use to denote that someone is a clinician. You may also encounter the term "behavioral health" provider, which is often interchangeable with "mental health."

A **counselor** is a somewhat interchangeable term for therapist, and some therapists prefer it. Sometimes the term "counselor" may indicate that the person is not licensed or working to become licensed, which you can always ask at any time. Licensure ensures that the person offering therapy is receiving ongoing continuing education training and is also overseen by a state board.

A **peer counselor/peer specialist/peer support** is someone who had a similar experience to the one for which they now provide support. A peer counselor is not required to have a degree in psychology. You can often access peer support in settings such as rape crisis centers, domestic violence shelters, partial hospitals, and drug and alcohol programs, where they are able to provide support to others based on their own experiences and growth.

A **case manager** is responsible for helping you with day-to-day matters such as applying for insurance or social services benefits, obtaining housing and employment, and scheduling and transporting to medical or mental health appointments. Every case management program has different guidelines about what services they provide. A case manager is not able to provide therapy but is helpful if you are experiencing difficult life circumstances such as poverty, unemployment, or a mental health crisis. Case managers can typically be found in community mental health settings, discussed on page 242.

A **mental health coach** is someone who provides support and feedback on matters related to mental health. Coaching is not currently a regulated field, so coaches may or may not have advanced degrees and certifications. If you are considering seeing a coach, you can ask them what qualifications and/or certifications they have if that is important to you.

The terms **"behavioral health consultant"** and **"mental health consultant"** are commonly used when mental health professionals work in specialized settings, such as primary care or substance treatment.

24

Barriers to Finding a Mental Health Professional

FINANCES

Paying for therapy is one of the biggest barriers you may face in finding good therapy. It's part of what prompted us to write this book, because we believe quality mental health information should be available to everyone.

Many therapists have left insurance companies because of low reimbursement rates and the high amounts of stress and paperwork associated with the insurance industry. While we wish there was a quick fix, it is a big issue that requires a systemic overhaul to correct. In the meantime, there are a few options that may help.

Community mental health (CMH) is often the name for the lowest-cost mental health resources in the US. If you do an online search for your city or county with the words "community mental health," you should find options near you. Community mental health is usually free or low cost if you are considered low income. You can usually receive medication management, therapy, and case management through a CMH agency. It is important to note that if you are seeking medication management through CMH, they will likely require you to see one of their therapists.

If you have been a victim of a crime in the US, you are likely to qualify for free therapy. This may be found at your local crime victims agency, such as a rape crisis center or domestic violence agency. If your local area does not have such an agency or if your need falls outside of their scope, you may be eligible to be reimbursed for counseling expenses elsewhere. In addition, some states have financial programs you can use if you were sexually abused in childhood, whether or not the crime was ever reported.

If you have limited financial resources and want to meet with a clinician, local graduate psychology programs will often provide low-cost therapy services. You meet with a masters- or doctoral-level student who is supervised by a licensed psychologist, social worker, LPC, etc. If you are a college student and your school has a counseling center, you can usually see a licensed clinician there for free.

Insurance is not accessible to everyone, and you may not have adequate mental health coverage even if you are insured. However, if you are insured, it's always worth calling your insurance company to see what therapists local to you accept your insurance. You can also search on some online therapist directories according to your insurance.

If your workplace offers an Employee Assistance Program (EAP), use it! Some plans will let you choose a therapist outside their network if the therapist will complete the associated EAP paperwork provided.

Some therapists offer sliding scale therapy (sessions with adjusted pricing according to income). See this chapter's Resources section for options.

While low-cost online therapy has proliferated in recent years, it's important to make an informed decision before signing up for a low-cost online therapy service. Some of the best-known platforms have faced major lawsuits due to their mishandling of sensitive client data, and others are known within the therapist community for having unethical onboarding processes that leave therapists without support and in precarious situations. Like with many online decisions, it's good to do your research and get recommendations for specific clinicians before signing up for an online service.

LACK OF ACCESS

If you live in a rural area or if your first language isn't English, accessing helpful therapy in your region or with a therapist who speaks your first language can be barrier. While you may be able to attend therapy in English, being able to discuss emotional topics in your first language often leads to a much better experience.

Virtual therapy or teletherapy (meeting with a therapist through a secure online video service), can help with this barrier, and studies suggest that teletherapy and in-person therapy are equally effective.[5] When you have the choice, choosing between teletherapy and in-person therapy is a personal decision. You may prefer in-person therapy for reasons such as being able to use art or somatic therapies in session, because it's important for you to be face-to-face with your therapist, if you have a trauma history related to the internet, or you lack privacy in your home making online therapy feel unsafe. Conversely, you may just as strongly prefer teletherapy because you can be in the safe, comfortable environment of your own home and to save time and money not having to travel.

You should choose the kind of therapy that feels the safest, most comfortable, and most confidential to you. Keep in mind that some therapy licenses require the therapist and you to be physically located, at the time of your appointment, in the same state where they are licensed.

A common reason why people stay with a therapist they know isn't right for them is the fear of hurting the therapist's feelings. A client may feel vulnerable in the therapeutic relationship, so it can be hard for them to say "You aren't the right therapist for me." However, leaving a stagnant, unhelpful, or even potentially harmful therapy relationship is a critical part of getting the support you need and finding success in therapy.

How to Break Up with a Therapist

When we worked with kids in therapy, we shared the true story of Balto to explain when it was time to move on. Balto was the lead sled dog that helped deliver diphtheria medication to the remote village of Nome, Alaska, in 1925, when the snow was too deep for anything other than a sled dog relay to save the villagers' lives. Many dog sled teams ran through blizzard conditions for almost six days to get the medication there in time. The teams passed the medication to each other at numerous stops along the way, until it finally reached Nome.

When it came time for children to be finished with therapy, we would explain to them that we were just one part of their "sled dog team," but that throughout their lives, it would take many teams, including family members, teachers, friends, and maybe other therapists to get them to where they need to go. Balto may be a children's story, but the principle applies to adults, too. It's normal that not just one therapist will get you all the way to your finish line. If you feel it's time to break up with a therapist or to ask for your sessions to change, you can start by saying, "It's time for me to move on and try a different kind of therapy/a different therapist/a different approach to therapy."

Make the conversation a place for growth. If you struggle to ask for what you need or to set boundaries, let the therapist know that you want their support in that area as you practice it in real time on the topic of how your therapy relationship is going.

If you have a hard time having these conversations in person, consider sending a text or email before your session, saying that this is what you want to talk about. You can also use this book! Consider taking it to a session and explaining that this chapter has got you thinking about changes you want to make, either about how your therapy sessions go or about who you see.

If a therapist doesn't react well to you setting boundaries, asking for something different, or changing therapists, it's only an indication that they're not the right therapist for you. However, many therapists will respond to this supportively, and will either make the changes you need or help you find a therapist who will be a better fit.

How to Communicate While Seeking a Mental Health Professional

IF YOU'RE THE ONE SEEKING A MENTAL HEALTH PROFESSIONAL

Don't give up! Finding the right therapist can be a daunting journey. Sometimes you have to go through several therapists before you finally find the one that is right for you.

We've shared ways to make sure your mental health professional is holding up their end of the deal, but make sure you do, too. Be completely honest with your therapist; even though this can be scary, it's the only way to make sure you are getting the right help. If you are attending virtual therapy, make sure to be in a safe, quiet, private location, not driving in your car or working on chores!

IF A LOVED ONE IS SEEKING A MENTAL HEALTH PROFESSIONAL

Often, people find the best therapist for them not from an internet search, but from recommendations from family and friends. If your loved one is trying to find a therapist, ask the people you know for recommendations.

But first, note that you shouldn't share who you're trying to find the therapist for. That's your loved one's business and should be kept confidential unless they want it shared. Instead, you can ask your connections for recommendations by saying something like, "I'm looking for a therapist for a friend who has anxiety/depression/sleep issues. Do you know of anyone?"

IF YOU'RE SEEKING A MENTAL HEALTH PROFESSIONAL FOR A CHILD

Make sure to connect with someone who specializes in working with children. You wouldn't bring your child to a medical professional who only sees adults, and you shouldn't do that with a mental health professional, either. There are numerous kinds of mental health treatment that work for children, but any mental health professional who works with kids should be fluent in the language of play in addition to the therapy modality (for example, Cognitive Behavioral Therapy or Parent-Child Interaction Therapy) they're trained to use. And while the therapist should still maintain the same ethical boundaries used with adults, your child should enjoy seeing them. Children should feel safe and cared for in therapy, although with professional boundaries in place. You can explain to your child that this is a time-limited helping relationship like the one they have with a teacher, and that they will eventually "graduate" from therapy. You can also use the Balto story to explain this to them.

If you're seeking mental health treatment for a teen, note that some states have laws about what age a child is entitled to mental health treatment without parental consent or involvement. In many states this age is fourteen. So, while your teen's mental health professional should not disclose information about them without their consent, it's still important for you to be involved in some way. Scheduling joint sessions for you and your teen is one of the best ways to make this happen. Many therapists will also involve you at the end of some sessions to ensure everyone stays on the same page, in addition to occasional family or parent/child sessions.

With this said, there are some situations in which the therapist will need to focus exclusively on developing a relationship with your teen in order to build trust and the therapeutic relationship. If the ultimate goal is for all of you to communicate when your teen is ready, let them take their time. Teenagers need increasing levels of autonomy and privacy, even though effective treatment must ultimately involve their caretakers, too.

What Finding the Right Mental Health Professional Can Look Like in Real Life

Devon has been in therapy for years, seeing the same therapist that they saw during a major life event. Over time the therapy has seemed like it's become less and less helpful. Sometimes Devon finds themself skipping sessions because they don't want to spend the money. Still, it feels hard to let their therapist go. After all, they were there for Devon during a really hard time, and they know them better than almost anyone. Devon worries that if they leave their therapist they won't have the support if they need it in the future.

After reading this book, Devon feels hopeful that maybe the therapist for the next stage of their journey is out there. They keep thinking about it all week, so before their next session they send their therapist a message that says, "I really appreciate all you've done for me. However, I'd like to try a new kind of therapy. I think this session should be our last one." Devon is so nervous when the day comes to go back to therapy, but to their surprise their therapist is supportive. They tell Devon that a termination session is an important part of successful therapy, so they spend the session celebrating Devon's progress over the years and brainstorming some things Devon wants to work on in the future. Devon feels good about the session, and it feels like the relationship ended well.

A couple of weeks later, they have consult calls with several different potential therapists. They go to an intake appointment, but while they are there the therapist says something that makes Devon feel misunderstood. Devon doesn't schedule a next appointment, and they think about giving up on the whole process, but they keep trying.

Devon searches a therapist directory for the specialization they're looking for. It takes a few consultations, but they find someone they feel safe with. Some weeks they just need to talk, and they always know the therapist isn't judging them. Other weeks they need help, and they leave with new insight and ideas to move forward. When Devon looks back, they feel proud of themself for making the change they needed and deserved.

READING LIST AND OTHER RESOURCES

Therapist directories are a great place to start your journey toward finding the right therapist for you. Here are some options.

Inclusive Therapists Directory (inclusivetherapists.com), Therapy Den (therapyden.com), and Deconstructing the Mental Health System (dmhsus.org/find-a-bipoc-therapist-or-healer) include therapists who specialize in working with marginalized communities or identify as marginalized persons themselves.

The Trauma Therapist Network (traumatherapistnetwork.com) can help you find therapists who are trauma-informed.

Therapy for Black Girls (therapyforblackgirls.com), Clinicians of Color (cliniciansofcolor.org), and Therapy for Black Men (therapyforblackmen.org) can help you find Black therapists.

The American Association of Christian Counselors (aacc.net) can help you find Christian therapists.

One Sky Center (oneskycenter.org) connects Indigenous people with evidence-based services.

Asian Mental Health Collective (asianmhc.org) and LatinX Therapy (latinxtherapy.com) list therapists who speak languages other than English.

National Queer and Trans Therapists of Color Network (nqttcn.com/en) list trans-informed and affirming therapists.

Vet Centers are a place to access evidence-based mental health care if you are a veteran.

The Open Path Collective (openpathcollective.org) features therapists who offer sliding scale therapy.

If you have been a victim of crime, you may be eligible for reimbursement for mental health treatment. Visit the Office for Victims of Crime for more information (ovc.ojp.gov/help-for-victims/help-in-your-state).

If you have the financial means, consider donating to a cause that offers sliding scale or scholarship pricing for others, such as The Loveland Foundation, Beauty after Bruises, or Open Path. You can also establish a scholarship with a local therapist whose work you believe in.

If you're looking for a therapist who is certified in a specific therapy modality, such as EMDR, TF-CBT, or IFS, many certification websites list the therapists trained in that model. (Please note that not every therapist who has specializations will be listed in a directory. Some directories have costs or other prohibitions that deter therapists from listing.)

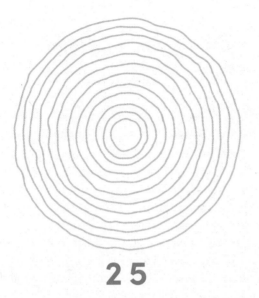

25

NAVIGATING PRIMARY CARE

You are not alone if you have sought support for mental health problems in primary care.[1] Primary care clinicians deliver a large and growing portion of frontline outpatient mental health care in the United States.[2]

You may encounter several collaborative care models that involve mental health clinicians (also called "behavioral health consultants" in primary care settings) working together with primary care clinicians, accessible as part of the care team. You may find that seeing a mental health clinician in the primary care setting is more convenient and may also reduce your stress around mental health stigma.[3] Collaborative care models are likely to have a beneficial impact on either an adult or child's mental health.[4] Whether or not your primary care office uses a collaborative care approach, it can be helpful to consider several factors when seeking treatment, including for mental health, in primary care.

How to Get More from Your Primary Care Appointments

MAKE SHARED DECISIONS ABOUT YOUR HEALTH

Shared decision-making involves you and a clinician sharing information, building a consensus about the preferred treatment, and agreeing on what treatment will be implemented.[5] When taking part in shared decision-making, it's important for clinicians to help you understand information by avoiding medical jargon, focusing on a few key topics during a visit, breaking down information or instructions into small concrete steps, and checking in with you to assess your understanding of what has been discussed.[6] When considering that primary care clinicians need to care for you from a biological, psychological, and social perspective, this can be more challenging.

The relationship between you and your clinician is a central factor in the making of health care decisions.[7] The SMART criteria, as set out by George Doran, can help you set specific, measurable, attainable, relevant, and time-bound goals. It's important to feel able to speak openly with your clinician about your goals and to let them know when a goal doesn't feel realistic for you. If you don't feel comfortable speaking in this way to your primary care clinician, it may be a sign to find a new one.

SET AN AGENDA

Set an agenda at the beginning of your appointment. Clinicians will often ask you to list all of the concerns that you would like to discuss. Even if they don't ask, it is often helpful if you provide them with the top concerns you are hoping to focus on.

Though it may seem counterintuitive, it can be helpful not to provide too much detail when listing your concerns. Clinicians may change their style of interaction and engage in less patient-centered communication depending on the number of agenda items you bring to a visit.[8] If you have only one topic to discuss, the conversation may be more collaborative, but less so if there are two to six agenda items due to the time constraints of the clinician's schedule.[9]

This may mean that it's actually more efficient for you to go to your primary care clinician more regularly so that you can discuss timely concerns, instead of saving them up for a once-yearly checkup.

WRITE DOWN THE TOPICS YOU'D LIKE TO DISCUSS

Especially if you need medication refills or paperwork completed, it's worth writing down the topics to discuss. It's often helpful to tell the nurse, after they've guided you to the exam room, the things you would like to discuss so they can communicate this with the primary care clinician on your behalf, so that they can be aware of it when you are both mutually setting the visit agenda.

THE RESEARCH SAYS . . .

You Are Not Alone

Health literacy is the ability to understand and apply health information, like signing consent forms, reading food and medicine labels, and applying for insurance. A 2003 study found that more than one third of American adults had limited health literacy.[11] If you have low health literacy, you are more likely to have poorer health outcomes and poorer use of health care services.[12]

FOLLOW THROUGH ON THE GOALS YOU SET

If you've worked with your primary care clinician to set goals for yourself, follow through on them. For example, you may be asked to keep a log of your blood sugar levels, blood pressure, or sleep patterns. This information helps the clinician to know the best evidence-based treatments to discuss with you, so give it your best effort to do this tracking when asked.

DISCUSS YOUR MENTAL HEALTH CONCERNS OPENLY

You're not alone if you experience mental health struggles. Your primary care clinician should be a safe person with whom you can confidentially share your concerns and receive care. They can often start mental health treatment (for example, discussing coping skills and medications), and refer you to additional support if needed.

If you are comfortable doing so, this can also include discussing your trauma history. Medical clinicians may have varying levels of experience with patients who have a history of childhood sexual or physical abuse, which may result in them perceiving the interactions to be more difficult.[10] Disclosing your trauma history can help your clinician understand and have compassion for why your case may be complicated.

Barriers to Having a Good Primary Care Relationship

DISCRIMINATION AND RACIAL BIAS

Discrimination and racial bias may be a barrier to fully engaging with your primary care clinician. Feelings of perceived discrimination can be a common barrier in health care appointments, especially if you're Black, Latinx/Hispanic, uninsured, or have a mental health diagnosis.[13]

Due to a long history of institutionalized racism in the United States, this is not an easy trauma history to overcome. If you find your anxiety or medical system–related stressors are getting in the way of you receiving medical care, it may be helpful to process this in therapy so that you can ultimately advocate for getting the medical care you need and deserve.

You do not need to tolerate a clinician who is discriminating against you, even unconsciously, because of your race or for any other reason. Research is clear that racial discrimination leads to poorer health outcomes,[14] even including death.[15] If the options for racially competent care in your area are limited, there may be a telehealth clinician available for some medical concerns.

STRESS AND ANXIETY ABOUT MEDICAL TREATMENT

You may feel stressed about going to see a clinician. If this avoidance is due to you having high levels of anxiety related to worrying about having or acquiring an illness, it could be a sign you have Illness Anxiety Disorder.[16]

With Illness Anxiety Disorder, you may either seek medical care often, or avoid it as much as possible. Avoidance maintains anxiety, so it's recommended to seek medical care routinely. If you have trauma related to medical appointments, check out page 151 for some specific strategies for coping with this.

MEDICAL COSTS

Costs such as loss of income during the appointment time, insurance premiums and copays, travel, and childcare could all be possible barriers to seeing your primary care clinician or following up on mental health recommendations.

Depending on your income, you may qualify for medical assistance. Some clinics are federally qualified health centers that serve an underserved area or population, offer sliding fee scales for patients, accept Medicaid and Medicare, and provide additional services such as mental health, dental, and other specialty care (either on-site or with another clinician/group). (For more information about finding a social worker or a case manager who may be able to help you access care, see chapter 22.)

SHORT TIME FRAMES FOR APPOINTMENTS

The short time frame afforded for primary care appointments, often around only fifteen to thirty minutes, and the time needed for clinicians to apply preventive and chronic disease care guidelines can leave little time for open dialogue and thorough discussions about your mental health.[17] Use your time wisely by bringing a list of your concerns and working with your clinician to set an agenda at the beginning of the appointment.

How to Communicate with Your Primary Care Clinician

IF YOU'RE THE ONE SEEKING MEDICAL CARE

Reach out to someone who supports you to see if they are willing to accompany you to your appointment. This could include them sitting in the waiting room or coming into the exam room with you. You can also reach out to the office in advance and let them know how they could increase your comfort level. This may include asking to be scheduled early to be the first person seen in a clinic session.

As much as possible, be open with your clinician about your agenda items and what you see as barriers to care. This can help you mutually set an agenda and provide opportunities for you to problem solve together to come up with a realistic treatment plan for your care.

25

NAVIGATING PRIMARY CARE

IF A LOVED ONE IS SEEKING MEDICAL CARE

Offer to go to an appointment with them, but don't pressure them into going, as this may cause them to feel more resistant. Encourage them to speak openly with their clinicians and give them the privacy to do so during their appointments.

IF YOU'RE SEEKING MEDICAL CARE FOR A CHILD

Preparing them for any medical appointments or tests using words they can understand is key. We all do better when stress is predictable, so letting your child know what to expect will help them cope. This also allows them to prepare and practice the coping strategies discussed throughout this book, such as breathing or grounding techniques.

What Navigating Primary Care Can Look Like in Real Life

Miguel lost insurance coverage as he was no longer able to stay on his parent's plan after the age of twenty-six. He was able to get new insurance coverage, but he has a high deductible and so he didn't plan to seek medical care if he could help it. Nevertheless, he started experiencing symptoms of depression and eventually decided that he would call his primary care office to make an appointment.

At the appointment, Miguel is taken to an exam room by a nurse, and they ask him questions about his mood. His clinician shares with him that based on the screening questionnaire he may meet criteria for major depression. He discusses his symptoms in more detail and it does seem likely that he has been experiencing episodes of depression.

The primary care clinician shares with Miguel that there are behavioral health consultants, mental health clinicians with experience providing care in primary care settings, that work in the clinic and if he has time, one could come meet with him for fifteen minutes at the end of his visit. He agrees and continues the appointment. He discusses possibly starting a medication for depression, and the primary care clinician asks if he would be willing to have some lab work completed to check for things that could impact his mood and to screen for general health factors like diabetes and cholesterol.

Miguel then meets with the behavioral health consultant and discusses the strategy of behavioral activation, which includes increasing his activity levels throughout the day even if he doesn't feel initially motivated to do so. He schedules a follow-up with both his primary care clinician and the behavioral health consultant. It's convenient because he can see them both at the same location on the same date.

During Miguel's follow-up to discuss his labs, he learns that his hemoglobin A1C, a measure of his average blood sugar level over the last three months, is high and he has prediabetes. Luckily there is also a diabetic educator who is part of the clinic care team, and they meet with him to discuss improvements he can make to his diet, to ensure he can have a healthier future.

READING LIST AND OTHER RESOURCES

The American Medical Association has a resource called "What Doctors Wish Patients Knew About Trauma-Informed Care" that can help inform you as a patient about what trauma-informed care looks like. You can find this by searching "What Doctors Wish Patients Knew About Trauma-Informed Care" on their website: ama-assn.org.

If you are a health care clinician, the California Health Care Foundation has an online tool kit to Advance Racial Health Equity in Primary Care: chcf.org/wp-content/uploads/2022/07/ToolkitRacialEquityPrimaryCareImprovement.pdf.

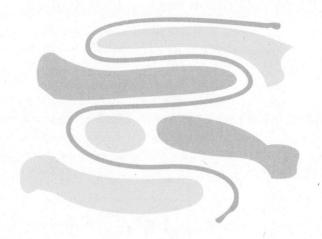

26

NAVIGATING INSURANCE AND SELF-PAY

D ealing with and understanding the ins and outs of how to find and pay for mental health treatment can be confusing and stressful, and even more so when you're simultaneously dealing with a mental or physical illness. In many cases, using your insurance to pay for mental health services, even if you have a copay or coinsurance, may be more affordable than paying out of pocket (also known as self-pay or private pay). Even with insurance, the cost of therapy may not be within your budget. Moreover, as tricky and costly as navigating insurance can be, there are millions of individuals in the US who do not have insurance coverage. In this chapter, we hope to give you some information and resources to help you navigate the mental health payment system.

A Quick Guide to Insurance and Therapy Terms

Knowing insurance and therapy lingo can help you understand your coverage and feel more confident in deducing what you're able to afford when it comes to seeking treatment. In addition, it's important to know what information your clinician is required to give to your insurance to ensure that your session is covered. Here, you'll find a list of some common insurance and therapy terms.

Benefit year: A benefit year is the entire twelve months of your insurance coverage. January 1 is the start of the benefit year for many insurances, although yours may begin during another month. Certain aspects of your policy, such as your deductible, will renew (or start over again) at the start of your benefit year.

Claim: In order to get paid for services provided to you, your clinician will submit a claim to your insurance, which includes your demographic information (such as name, address, gender, and date of birth), date of service, time that service took place, length of your session, and your diagnosis/diagnoses.

Coinsurance: This is the percentage of your treatment's cost that you're responsible for paying once you've met your deductible. For example, your coinsurance for therapy sessions may be 10 percent, meaning you're responsible for paying 10 percent of the total cost. This varies from having a set copay cost, as the amount you owe depends on what the insurance has agreed to pay your clinician for the therapy services provided to you.

Copay: A set amount that you need to pay for each session, aside from deductibles or coinsurance. If your

THE RESEARCH SAYS . . .

You Are Not Alone

About 7 percent of US residents of all ages were uninsured in the first quarter of 2023.[1] Almost 25 percent of adults with a mental illness report that they have been unable to connect with the mental health services they desperately need.[2] This is partly due to having no or inadequate insurance coverage, the lack of available clinicians, and limited financial ability to pay out of pocket for services.[3]

copay is twenty-five dollars per session, that is what you'll be expected to pay each time you meet with your mental health clinician.

Deductible: The annual amount you have to pay out of pocket before your insurance begins to cover the service you're seeking. If you have a $1,500 deductible, that means you'll have to pay $1,500 out of pocket before your insurance pays for some or all of the service. Therefore, you'll be responsible for the full cost of each session until you've met the deductible.

Diagnosis: Insurance companies require that you be given a diagnosis (for example, Major Depressive Disorder or Panic Disorder) to determine if your therapy sessions will be covered. This diagnosis may become part of your permanent medical and insurance records. If you apply for life insurance, you may be asked for your past history of diagnoses and to provide your medical records. You may opt to restrict information that your insurance company has access to, such as your diagnosis, although this may result in your sessions not being covered.

If your insurance audits your clinician's records, which is often done to ensure the medical necessity of sessions and that the clinician is keeping all the necessary records, your insurance may have access to your detailed medical record (for example, notes about your sessions and goals for treatment).

If you choose the self-pay route or need to use this due to not having insurance, you may not be given a diagnosis by your clinician as the requirements of insurance do not apply. It's also possible the reason you are seeking therapy may not be something that falls within the criteria of a diagnosis. Your life and mood might be pretty good, and you may just want to work on setting boundaries. However, if you are seeking reimbursement from your insurance for your sessions, they may require a diagnosis before providing that reimbursement.

Employee Assistance Program: Some employers offer Employee Assistance Programs (EAPs), which cover the cost of therapy for a limited number of sessions. These session limits are usually shorter than what insurance offers, such as four to six sessions.

Explanation of benefit: The Explanation of Benefit (EOB) is a letter you receive from your insurance company detailing the date you received your therapy service, the amount billed by your clinician, how much your insurance paid your clinician, and how much you owe.

Good Faith Estimate (GFE): A Good Faith Estimate is your right as a mental (or physical) health consumer since the Federal No Surprises Act that went into effect on January 1, 2023. This estimate gives you a snapshot of what you may pay, if you are uninsured or doing self-pay, if you were to meet weekly with your clinician within a certain time period (for example, one year) or within the format that your services are provided (such as a five-day trauma intensive program). You should automatically receive a GFE from your mental health clinician, but if you don't, you can request one. Your GFE should include your estimated payment amount, and also information on how to file a dispute if you are charged the wrong amount.

Often, it can be difficult to determine how much time you'll actually be in therapy, as this is dependent on your individual needs, but a GFE can provide some insight into what financial investment you may be making in your mental and emotional health.

You may find more information on this at cms.gov/nosurprises.

In-network provider: This is a clinician who accepts your insurance. Of note, "provider" is an insurance term for a clinician. Throughout this book, we use the term "clinician" as it is a more person-focused term.

Opting out of your insurance: For many reasons, you may not want to use your insurance for your sessions even though the therapist you want to work with accepts it. Sometimes, it's more affordable not to use your insurance or you may not want your insurance to have a record of your therapy sessions. In this case, you may be asked to sign an "opt-out form" stating that you are choosing not to use your coverage for sessions.

Out-of-network provider: This is a clinician who doesn't accept your insurance. If you choose to see an out-of-network provider, you may need to pay for your sessions out of pocket.

Reimbursement: If you have to pay out of pocket to see an out-of-network provider, depending on your insurance coverage, you may be eligible to be reimbursed for some percentage of what you paid for your therapy session(s).

If you would like to submit for reimbursement, ask your clinician for a superbill (see definition on the next page) for you to submit directly to your insurance or through a third-party service.

Self-pay: Also known as private pay, self-pay means you pay the full amount for the session out of pocket. You can do this regardless of whether you have insurance.

Session limit: Your insurance may cover only a certain number of therapy sessions, say thirty sessions, during a calendar or benefit year; this is known as your session limit. If you're meeting with your clinician weekly, this is important information to know.

Sliding scale: Some clinicians offer sliding scale or pro bono sessions if you are financially limited. Sliding scale is often based on your yearly income or what you're able to afford.

Superbill: A superbill is a detailed receipt of the services you received from a clinician.

Strategies for More Effectively Navigating Insurance

BE INFORMED

Even if your clinician or clinician's office informs you of your financial responsibility and coverage details, it is important for you to contact your insurance company yourself to make sure you have accurate information and understand your coverage.

Some questions you might want to ask your insurance company include the following.

- Do I have mental/behavioral health insurance benefits? (This is important to know as mental health coverage can be separate from physical health coverage, similar to eye and dental insurance coverage.)

- Is there a deductible? If yes, what is my deductible? Has it been met? What percentage am I responsible for paying (the coinsurance) after it has been met?

- Do I have a copay? How much is it?

- How many visits per year are covered? (This will tell you what your session limit is.)

- What are the dates of my benefit year?
- Which services are covered (telehealth, couples therapy . . .)?
- If I'm having telehealth sessions, do they need to be on a certain telehealth platform?
- Do I need a pre-authorization?

Some questions you might want to ask your clinician include the following.

- Do you accept [my insurance]? (In insurance terms, "Are you an in-network provider/clinician with my insurance?")
- What is your contracted rate? (Ask this if you have a deductible. Essentially, you are asking, "What do I have to pay for each session?")
- Do you offer a sliding scale? (This is if you are unable to afford your copay, deductible, coinsurance, or self-pay rate. Also inquire whether there is a time limit for the sliding scale. Clinicians will likely ask for proof of your income, which could be a paycheck or last year's tax returns. Some clinicians will only offer a sliding scale for a certain number of sessions.)

Barriers to Effectively Navigating Insurance

PRICE

High monthly premiums, deductibles, and copays can make it challenging to afford any type of treatment, particularly mental health treatment. As you often start treatment by meeting your clinician on a weekly basis, these costs can add up.

CONFUSING POLICIES

There can be so many details when it comes to insurance that it can be difficult to understand what's actually covered. We encourage you to ask questions until you get the clarity that you need.

EXCLUDED SERVICES

Some policies do not cover certain services, such as couples therapy or diagnostic assessment (testing) for certain diagnoses, such as ADHD. These exclusions can be barriers to seeking the care that you may need, particularly if your finances are limited and you're unable to pay out of pocket.

LACK OF CLINICIANS WHO ACCEPT YOUR INSURANCE

Due to the restrictions of many insurance companies and limited reimbursement to clinicians, many clinicians do not accept insurance and instead, only accept self-pay. This means that the pool of in-network clinicians may be limited in your area. It is sometimes easier to connect with a clinician who accepts self-pay, although that is a privilege that many do not have.

It can be frustrating if a clinician does not accept your insurance and their self-pay hourly rates are too high for you. It is valid to feel frustrated. These rates may seem more understandable when considering that there are many costs for clinicians that are not as obvious. Clinicians need to pay for their malpractice insurance, liability insurance, health insurance, income taxes, telehealth platform, electronic health record, phone line, online calendar, website, annual professional license fees, annual continuing education credits for their license, professional memberships, board certification, business licenses, licenses to practice in multiple states, and so on. If they practice in person, they are likely paying rent and utility bills. Many therapists are also making high student loan payments in order to pay off their debt from the graduate degree(s) required for their license.

How to Communicate About Insurance

IF YOU'RE THE ONE NAVIGATING INSURANCE AND SELF-PAY

Insurance can be helpful and a pain all at once. It may afford more opportunities for receiving care, although the confusion around what is actually covered may stop you from taking full advantage of it. If you're finding yourself feeling confused or overwhelmed, please reach out to a loved one or call a customer service representative at your insurance company and ask questions to clarify what's covered. (See page 260 for some helpful questions to start.)

IF A LOVED ONE IS NAVIGATING INSURANCE AND SELF-PAY

Be an advocate as much as you can. Keep in mind that it can be hard for someone to navigate insurance on their best day, and it can feel near impossible to navigate insurance on those less-than-great days when even getting out of bed feels hard.

Ask your loved one, "Would you like me to be there as you make the call to your insurance?" or say, "If you give permission for me to talk to them, I'll be happy to do so. We can even be on speaker phone so you can also hear what they say."

Some mental health diagnoses, such as dissociative disorders or ADHD, may make it more difficult for your loved one to remember what the health insurance representative told them. If they would like you to do so, listen in on the call and help them take notes, as well as remind them what was said.

What Dealing with Insurance Can Look Like in Real Life

Alex connects with a clinician, and finds that their deductible applies to their therapy sessions. After Alex meets their deductible, then their coinsurance goes into effect. This means that they will have to pay what is called the clinician's contracted amount until they meet their deductible, which is the amount that their insurance has agreed to pay the clinician for services rendered to them.

Alex has a $2,500 deductible, their clinician's contracted rate is $100, and they have a 10 percent coinsurance after their deductible is met. That means Alex will be paying $100 per session until their deductible has been met. Since Alex doesn't have any other medical or mental health appointments they have to pay for, that means they end up paying $100 per session for twenty-five sessions, or about six months of weekly sessions, until their deductible is met. After their deductible is met, Alex is responsible for 10 percent of the session cost, which means they're now paying $10 per session. Sessions just got a lot more affordable! This new cost per session will remain in place until the start of Alex's next benefit year, at which point their deductible starts over.

Reimbursify.com is a website and app that you can use to submit for reimbursement from your insurance company for out-of-network services. A small fee may apply. (Reimbursement requests can also be submitted directly to your insurance company, typically through their website and/or your personal benefits page.)

Centers for Medicare and Medicaid Services (CMS) created the following resource to help navigate insurance coverage: cms.gov/priorities/health-equity/c2c#navigate-coverage.

Children may be eligible for low-cost coverage through the Children's Health Insurance Program (CHIP). CHIP includes free well visits and dental appointments for children, but other benefits vary by state. Find out your eligibility by calling 1-800-318-2596 (TTY: 1-855-889-4325) or filling out an application through the Health Insurance Marketplace.

For more resources, see page 248.

5

GETTING SUPPORT

GLOSSARY

Ableism is the discrimination and social prejudice against those with physical, intellectual, or mental disabilities. Historically, much value has been placed on social constructs of what is considered "normal" and "intelligent" and anything different from that has often been viewed as inferior. Something as common as the aging process has also been devalued, as it may impact your ability to navigate the world as you once did. If you don't live with a disability, you are considered to be able-bodied.

Acceptance and Commitment Therapy (ACT) involves reducing avoidance by processing your thoughts and feelings through use of acceptance, mindfulness, and values.

Attachment trauma results from insecure attachments in childhood, including infancy. While the events themselves may or may not seem traumatic at the time, they interrupt the important process of forming secure attachment, which is critical in setting you up for success in life. Like all trauma, Attachment Trauma may result from events, but commonly happens because what should have occurred *did not* occur. Attachment Trauma is often used interchangeably with Developmental Trauma.

Biopsychosocial model is an approach in which your clinicians will treat you as a whole person, considering the biological, psychological, and social factors that may impact your care.

Cisgender refers to you if your gender identity aligns with the biological sex you were assigned at birth.

Clinician is a professional who is qualified to practice medicine, psychology, or other allied health professions.

Cognitive Behavioral Therapy (CBT) is an effective treatment approach to manage a variety of mental health disorders. In this approach, your therapist will help you to identify and change the thoughts, feelings, and behaviors that may be keeping you stuck, to empower you.

Cognitive Behavioral Therapy for Insomnia (CBT-I) is an effective treatment for insomnia where you are guided to change sleep-related behaviors, with the focus on addressing conditioned arousal, ineffective sleep habits, and decreasing sleep-related worry.

Cognitive Processing Therapy (CPT) is a form of therapy for PTSD that involves similar cognitive strategies to CBT, and also strategies to allow you to reprocess and make new meaning of your experience of trauma.

Complex Post-Traumatic Stress Disorder (C-PTSD) is a diagnosis that is usually applied to people who have experienced childhood trauma, and who have symptoms of Developmental or Attachment Trauma in addition to the typical PTSD symptoms.

Dialectical Behavioral Therapy (DBT) is a form of psychotherapy based on Cognitive Behavioral Therapy (CBT), with special emphasis on learning to tolerate distress, which can be especially helpful if you have difficulty regulating your emotions. "Dialectical" means being able to understand and accept two things being true at once, such as that you are not responsible for the fact that you are suffering, but you are responsible for healing your suffering instead of enacting it on others.

Emotionally Focused Therapy (EFT) is an effective approach in helping individuals, couples, and families build emotional regulation skills and explore their attachment styles. It is a space to create safe emotional connections with each other and within themselves, with the goal of both reducing and better managing conflict.

Eye Movement Desensitization and Reprocessing (EMDR) is a model of trauma treatment that helps you reconsolidate your trauma memories in order to feel relief, and to find new meaning from your trauma experience. Using a form of bilateral stimulation such as eye movements or audio to activate your memory networks, the therapist will guide you through targeting and processing each of your trauma memories. EMDR takes places over eight phases, and each phase may last anywhere from a few sessions to several months depending on your trauma history.

    Adjunctive EMDR is when you participate in EMDR with an EMDR-certified therapist, while also continuing your regular therapy with your primary therapist. Sometimes adjunctive EMDR is done in an intensive EMDR setting, where you complete it in a few days or weeks of repeated sessions.

Illness Anxiety Disorder, also known as hypochondriasis or health anxiety, is excessive worry that you have or will develop an illness or undiagnosed medical condition.

Imposter phenomenon, or imposter syndrome, is the experience of questioning your intelligence, skills, and abilities, feeling like a fraud, and the inability to fully recognize your accomplishments.

Internal Family Systems Therapy (IFS) is a form of therapy that helps you connect to your parts of self and begin to unburden them through connecting with the core self (which according to IFS is the part of self never harmed by trauma called "the natural healing agent of the system").

Medication-Assisted Treatment (MAT) is the use of medications along with behavioral therapy in the treatment of substance use disorders.

Neurofeedback, a type of biofeedback, includes use of an electroencephalography (EEG) to obtain information about your brainwave activity and provide you with real-time feedback, so you may try to influence the activity.

Obsessive-Compulsive Disorder (OCD) results in the experience of either or both: uncontrollable and recurrent thoughts, urges, or images (obsessions), and engagement in repetitive behaviors or mental acts in an effort to prevent or reduce a dreaded event (compulsions).

Perfectionism is when you place unrealistic standards on yourself (such as to never make a mistake) and often engage in damaging, self-critical talk.

Persistent Depressive Disorder includes experiencing a depressed mood most of the day, for more days than not, for at least two years (or one year for a child). While depressed, you experience at least two of the following symptoms: insomnia or hypersomnia, low energy/fatigue, low self-esteem, poor appetite/overeating, poor concentration or difficulty making decisions, or feelings of hopelessness.

Polyvagal theory explores the way the nervous system functions. The concept of coregulation comes from polyvagal theory.

Primary attachments are the caregivers that shape a child's world, first in utero with their biological mother, and then the people who are responsible for the child after birth, whether biological or adoptive parents, grandparents, or other important caregivers. These are the people who, first and foremost, make a child feel either safe or unsafe in the world.

Somatic therapy aims to bring healing to the body (known in Greek as "soma") as well as the mind, using the mind-body connection. Some examples of somatic therapies are somatic experiencing, sensorimotor therapy, and neurofeedback.

Sensorimotor psychotherapy is a kind of somatic therapy designed to treat PTSD. It integrates movement into traditional talk therapy to help you develop the internal resources to regulate your nervous system and heal the impact of trauma on the body.

Somatic experiencing was developed to help people move their trauma responses through their body instead of being stuck in a freeze, fight, flight, or fawn response. It uses awareness of physical sensations, developing connection with the body, and movement.

Trauma can be defined in many ways, but essentially it is an experience that overwhelms our brain and body's usual abilities to cope. Trauma is sometimes thought of as "too much, too fast," such as in an assault or a natural disaster, or "too little, too long," such as neglect or abandonment.

Some people like to use the terms "big T trauma" and "little t trauma." These terms are not meant to minimize or elevate one form of trauma over the other; instead, we can think of "big T trauma" as explosive events and "little t trauma" as erosive events. Both explosion and erosion have the power to change us.

Trauma-Focused Cognitive Behavioral Therapy (TF-CBT) helps you learn about your experience of trauma and learn new coping strategies, as well as create and process a trauma narrative about your experience, which is a guided way to express the story of your trauma through writing, art, or other creative ways. TF-CBT is particularly helpful for children who have experienced trauma.

Trauma-Sensitive Yoga (TSY) is a form of yoga that gives you total choice and control over how you want to move your body as you are healing from trauma. Unlike prescriptive yoga, TSY helps you get in touch with your body and what you need in a gentle way and on your own time. For more, check out traumasensitiveyoga.com.

NOTES

Introduction

1. Roberts, K. M., and A. N. Trejo, "Provider, Heal Thy System: An Examination of Institutionally Racist Healthcare Regulatory Practices and Structures," *Contemporary Family Therapy* 44, no. 1 (2022): 4–15.
2. Naicker, R., and D. Nunan, "Racial Bias," Catalogue of Bias, catalogofbias.org/biases/racial-bias. Accessed May 7, 2024.
3. Goyal, D., et al, "Scoping Review of Racial and Ethnic Representation of Participants in Mental Health Research Conducted in the Perinatal Period During the COVID-19 Pandemic," *Journal of Obstetric, Gynecologic, and Neonatal Nursing* 52, no. 2 (2023): 117–27.
4. Hattery, A. J., et al., "Diversity, Equity, and Inclusion in Research Teams: The Good, The Bad, and The Ugly," *Race and Justice* 12 (2022): 505–30.

1. Depression

1. American Psychiatric Association, *Diagnostic and Statistical Manual of Mental Disorders, Fifth Edition, Text Revision* (Washington, DC: American Psychiatric Association Publishing, 2022).
2. Ramanuj, P., et al., "Depression in primary care: part 2—management," *BMJ* 365 (2019).
3. Furukawa, T. A., et al., "Initial treatment choices to achieve sustained response in major depression: a systematic review and network meta-analysis," *World Psychiatry* 20, no. 3 (2021): 387–96.
4. Schwartz, J., et al., "Ketamine for treatment-resistant depression: recent developments and clinical applications," *Evidence-Based Mental Health* 19 (2016): 35–38.
5. Ramanuj et al., op. cit.
6. Santoft, F., et al., "Cognitive behaviour therapy for depression in primary care: systematic review and meta-analysis," *Psychological Medicine* 49, no. 8 (2019): 1266–74.
7. Ramanuj et al., op. cit.
8. Kuroda, N., et al., "Discovering Common Elements of Empirically Supported Self-Help Interventions for Depression in Primary Care: A Systematic Review," *Journal of General Internal Medicine* 36, no. 4 (2021): 869–80.
9. Nezu, A. M., et al., *Problem-Solving Therapy: A Treatment Manual* (New York: Springer, 2013).
10. Markowitz, J. C., and M. M. Weissman, "Interpersonal psychotherapy: principles and applications," *World Psychiatry* 3, no. 3 (2004): 136–39.
11. Stern, R. S., et al., "Repairing attachment in families with depressed adolescents: A task analysis," *Journal of Clinical Psychology* 79, no. 1 (2023): 201–9.
12. "Depression and Other Common Mental Disorders: Global Health Estimates," World Health Organization, 2017, iris.who.int/bitstream/handle/10665/254610/WHO-MSD-MER-2017.2-eng.pdf?sequence=1&isAllowed=y. Accessed May 7, 2024.
13. Mokdad, A. H., et al., "The State of US Health, 1990–2016: Burden of Diseases, Injuries, and Risk Factors among US States," *JAMA* 319, no. 14 (2018): 1444–72.
14. Twenge, J. M., and T. E. Joiner, "U.S. Census Bureau-assessed prevalence of anxiety and depressive symptoms in 2019 and during the 2020 COVID-19 pandemic," *Depression and Anxiety* 37, no. 10 (2020): 954–56.
15. Hu, M. X., et al., "Exercise interventions for the prevention of depression: a systematic review of meta-analyses," *BMC Public Health* 20 (2020): 1255.
16. Pjrek, E., et al., "The Efficacy of Light Therapy in the Treatment of Seasonal Affective Disorder: A Meta-Analysis of Randomized Controlled Trials," *Psychotherapy and Psychosomatics* 89, no. 1 (2020): 17–24.
17. Liang, Li, et al., "Latent profiles and transitions of daily routine disruptions are associated with severity of symptoms of anxiety and depression," *Leisure Sciences* (2023).

18. Elmer, T., and C. Stadtfeld, "Depressive symptoms are associated with social isolation in face-to-face interaction networks," *Scientific Reports* 10, no. 1 (2020).

19. Beck, J. S., *Cognitive Behavior Therapy: Basics and Beyond*, 3rd edition (New York: Guilford Press, 2020).

20. Chiriță, A. L., et al., "Current understanding of the neurobiology of major depressive disorder," *Romanian Journal of Morphology and Embryology* 56, suppl. 2 (2015): 651–58.

Krishnan, V., and E. J. Nestler, "The molecular neurobiology of depression," *Nature* 455, no. 7215 (2008): 894–902.

Yang, L., et al., "The effects of psychological stress on depression," *Current Neuropharmacology* 13, no. 4 (2015): 494–504.

21. Boswell, J. F., "Intervention strategies and clinical process in trans-diagnostic cognitive-behavioral therapy," *Psychotherapy* 50, no. 3 (2013): 381–86.

22. Boswell, J. F., et al., "Behavioral activation strategies in cognitive-behavioral therapy for anxiety disorders," *Psychotherapy* 54, no. 3 (2017): 231–36.

23. Lewinsohn, P. M., et al., "Behavioral treatment of depression," in P. O. Davidson (ed.), *The Behavioral Management of Anxiety, Depression, and Pain* (New York: Brunner/Mazel, 1976): 91–146.

24. Kuroda et al., op. cit.

25. Thaipisuttikul, P., et al., "Psychiatric comorbidities in patients with major depressive disorder," *Neuropsychiatric Disease and Treatment* 10 (2014): 2097–103.

26. "Mental Health by the Numbers," National Alliance on Mental Illness, nami.org/mhstats. Accessed May 7, 2024.

2. Anxiety

1. "Depression and Other Common Mental Disorders: Global Health Estimates," World Health Organization, 2017, iris.who.int/bitstream/handle/10665/254610/WHO-MSD-MER-2017.2-eng.pdf?sequence=1&isAllowed=y. Accessed May 7, 2024.

2. "Anxiety Disorders," National Institute of Mental Health, nimh.nih.gov/health/topics/anxiety-disorders. Accessed May 7, 2024.

3. Endler, N. S., and N. L. Kocovski, "State and trait anxiety revisited," *Journal of Anxiety Disorders* 15, no. 3 (2001): 231–45.

Spielberger, C. D., et al., *Manual for the State-Trait Anxiety Inventory (STAI)* (Palo Alto: Consulting Psychologists Press, 1983).

4. Limburg, K., et al., "The relationship between perfectionism and psychopathology: A meta-analysis," *Journal of Clinical Psychology* 73, no. 10 (2017): 1301–26.

5. Curran, T., and A. P. Hill, "Perfectionism is Increasing Over Time: A Meta-Analysis of Birth Cohort Differences from 1989 to 2016," *Psychological Bulletin* 145, no. 4 (2016): 410–29.

6. Kaczkurkin, A. N., and E. B. Foa, "Cognitive-Behavioral Therapy for Anxiety Disorders: An Update on the Empirical Evidence," *Dialogues in Clinical Neuroscience* 17, no. 3 (2015): 337–46.

7. Terlizzi, E. P., and M. A. Villarroel, "Symptoms of generalized anxiety disorder among adults: United States, 2019," *NCHS Data Brief*, no. 378 (2020): 1–8.

8. Ibid.

Remes, O., et al., "A systematic review of reviews on the prevalence of anxiety disorders in adult populations," *Brain and Behavior* 6, no. 7 (2016).

9. Vos, T., et al., "Global, Regional, and National Incidence, Prevalence, and Years Lived with Disability for 328 Diseases and Injuries for 195 Countries, 1990–2016: A Systematic Analysis for the Global Burden of Disease Study 2016," *The Lancet* 390, no. 10100 (2017): 1211–59.

10. Mokdad, A. H., et al., "The State of US Health, 1990–2016: Burden of Diseases, Injuries, and Risk Factors among US States," *JAMA* 319, no. 14 (2018): 1444–72.

11. Beck, J. S., *Cognitive Behavior Therapy: Basics and Beyond* (New York: Guilford Publications, 2020).

12. Vonderlin, R., et al., "Mindfulness-Based Programs in the Workplace: A Meta-Analysis of Randomized Controlled Trials," *Mindfulness* 11 (2020): 1579–98.

13. Liu, S., et al. "Sensorimotor rhythm neurofeedback training relieves anxiety in healthy people," *Cognitive Neurodynamics* 16 (2022): 531–44.

14. Mobbs, D., et al., "When fear is near: threat imminence elicits prefrontal-periaqueductal gray shifts in humans," *Science* 317, no. 5841 (2007): 1079–83.

Takagi, Y., et al. "A common brain network among state, trait, and pathological anxiety from whole-brain functional connectivity," *Neuroimage* 172 (2018): 506–16.

15. Daviu, N., et al., "Neurobiological links between stress and anxiety," *Neurobiology of Stress* 11 (2019): 100191.

16. Kabat-Zinn, J., *Wherever You Go, There You Are: Mindfulness Meditation in Everyday Life*, 30th Anniversary Edition (New York: Hachette, 2023).

17. Hopper, S. I., et al., "Effectiveness of Diaphragmatic Breathing for Reducing Physiological and Psychological Stress in Adults: A Quantitative Systematic Review," *JBI Database of Systematic Reviews and Implementation Reports* 17, no. 9 (2019): 1855–76.

18. Gerritsen, R. J. S., and G. P. H. Band, "Breath of Life: The Respiratory Vagal Stimulation Model of Contemplative Activity," *Frontiers in Human Neuroscience* 12 (2018): 397.

19. Neff, K., and C. Germer, "The Role of Self-Compassion in Psychotherapy," *World Psychiatry* 21, no. 1 (2022): 58–59.

20. Vos et al., op. cit.

21. Voss, P., et al., "Dynamic Brains and the Changing Rules of Neuroplasticity: Implications for Learning and Recovery," *Frontiers in Psychology* 8 (2017): 1657.

22. Akram, U., et al., "Dysfunctional Sleep-Related Cognition and Anxiety Mediate the Relationship Between Multidimensional Perfectionism and Insomnia Symptoms," *Cognitive Processing* 21, no. 1 (2020): 141–48.

Lamers, F., et al., "Comorbidity Patterns of Anxiety and Depressive Disorders in a Large Cohort Study: The Netherlands Study of Depression and Anxiety (NESDA)," *The Journal of Clinical Psychiatry* 72, no. 3 (2011): 341–48.

Batelaan, N., et al., "Panic Attacks as a Dimension of Psychopathology: Evidence for Associations with Onset and Course of Mental Disorders and Level of Functioning," *The Journal of Clinical Psychiatry* 73, no. 9 (2012): 1195–202.

23. Mitchell, A. J., et al., "Depression and Anxiety in Long-term Cancer Survivors Compared with Spouses and Healthy Controls: A Systematic Review and Meta-analysis," *Lancet Oncology* 14, no. 8 (2013): 721–32.

Molyneaux, E., et al., "Obesity and Mental Disorders During Pregnancy and Postpartum: A Systematic Review and Meta-analysis," *Obstetrics & Gynecology* 123, no. 4 (2014): 857–67.

Yang, Y. L., et al., "The Prevalence of Depression and Anxiety Among Chinese Adults with Cancer: A Systematic Review and Meta-analysis," *BMC Cancer* 13 (2013): 393.

3. Generalized Anxiety Disorder

1. American Psychiatric Association, *Diagnostic and Statistical Manual of Mental Disorders, Fifth Edition, Text Revision* (Washington, DC: American Psychiatric Association Publishing, 2022).

2. Remes, O., et al., "A Systematic Review of Reviews on the Prevalence of Anxiety Disorders in Adult Populations," *Brain and Behavior* 6, no. 7 (2016): e00497.

3. Andrews, G., et al., "Royal Australian and New Zealand College of Psychiatrists Clinical Practice Guidelines for the Treatment of Panic Disorder, Social Anxiety Disorder and Generalised Anxiety Disorder," *Australian & New Zealand Journal of Psychiatry* 52, no. 12 (2018): 1109–72.

"Generalised Anxiety Disorder and Panic Disorder in Adults: Management," National Institute for Health and Care Excellence, June 15, 2020, nice.org.uk/guidance/cg113/resources/generalised-anxiety-disorder-and-panic-disorder-in-adults-management-pdf-35109387756997.

Cuijpers, P., et al., "Psychological Treatment of Generalized Anxiety Disorder: A Meta-Analysis," *Clinical Psychology Review* 34, no. 2 (2014): 130–40.

4. Carpenter, J. K., et al., "Cognitive Behavioral Therapy for Anxiety and Related Disorders: A Meta-Analysis of Randomized Placebo-Controlled Trials," *Depression and Anxiety* 35, no. 6 (2018): 502–14.

5. Wilson, E. J., et al., "The Impact of Psychological Treatment on Intolerance of Uncertainty in Generalized Anxiety Disorder: A Systematic Review and Meta-Analysis," *Journal of Anxiety Disorders* 97 (2023): 102729.

6. Craske, M. G., and D. H. Barlow, *Mastery of Your Anxiety and Worry*, 2nd edition (New York: Oxford University Press, 2006).

7. Ji, J. L., et al., "Mental Imagery in Psychiatry: Conceptual & Clinical Implications," *CNS Spectrums* 24, no. 1 (2019): 114–26.

Penninx, B., et al., "Anxiety Disorders," *The Lancet* 397, no. 10277 (2021): 914–27.

8. Grossman, P., et al., "Mindfulness-Based Stress Reduction and Health Benefits: A Meta-Analysis," *Journal of Psychosomatic Research* 57, no. 1 (2004): 35–43.

9. "Generalised Anxiety Disorder and Panic Disorder," op. cit.

10. Szuhany, K. L., and N. M. Simon, "Anxiety Disorders: A Review," *JAMA* 328, no. 24 (2022): 2431–45.

11. LeDoux, J., and N. D. Daw, "Surviving Threats: Neural Circuit and Computational Implications of a New Taxonomy of Defensive Behaviour," *Nature Reviews Neuroscience* 19, no. 5 (2018): 269–82.

12. Alnaser, M. Z., et al., "Manifestation of Generalized Anxiety Disorder and Its Association with Somatic Symptoms Among Occupational and Physical Therapists During the COVID-19 Pandemic," *Frontiers in Public Health* 10 (2022): 891276.

13. Kumari, D., and J. Patil, "Guided Imagery for Anxiety Disorder: Therapeutic Efficacy and Changes in Quality of Life," *Industrial Psychiatry Journal* 32, suppl. 1 (2023): S191–95.

14. Fitzgerald, M., and M. Langevin, "Imagery," in R. Lindquist et al. (eds.), *Complementary and Alternative Therapies in Nursing: Mind-Body-Spirit-Therapies*, 7th edition (New York: Springer Publishing, 2014), 73–98.

15. Lemay, V., et al., "Impact of a Yoga and Meditation Intervention on Students' Stress and Anxiety Levels," *American Journal of Pharmaceutical Education* 83, no. 5 (2019): 7001.

16. Sugawara, A., et al., "Effects of Interoceptive Training on Decision Making, Anxiety, and Somatic Symptoms," *BioPsychoSocial Medicine* 14, no. 1 (2020): 7.

17. Szuhany and Simon, op. cit.

18. Stein, M. B., and J. Sareen, "Clinical Practice. Generalized Anxiety Disorder," *The New England Journal of Medicine* 373, no. 21 (2015): 2059–68.

19. Borza, L., "Cognitive-Behavioral Therapy for Generalized Anxiety," *Dialogues in Clinical Neuroscience* 19, no. 2 (2017): 203–8.

4. Social Anxiety

1. American Psychiatric Association, *Diagnostic and Statistical Manual of Mental Disorders, Fifth Edition, Text Revision* (Washington, DC: American Psychiatric Association Publishing, 2022).

2. Kessler, R. C., et al., "Lifetime Prevalence and Age-of-Onset Distributions of DSM-IV Disorders in the National Comorbidity Survey Replication," *Archives of General Psychiatry* 62, no. 6 (2005): 593–602.

3. Scaini, S., et al., "A Comprehensive Meta-Analysis of Cognitive-Behavioral Interventions for Social Anxiety Disorder in Children and Adolescents," *Journal of Anxiety Disorders* 42 (2016): 105–12.

4. Hofmann, S. G., "Cognitive Factors that Maintain Social Anxiety Disorder: A Comprehensive Model and its Treatment Implications," *Cognitive and Behavioral Therapy* 36, no. 4 (2007): 193–209.

5. Carpenter, J. K., et al., "Cognitive Behavioral Therapy for Anxiety and Related Disorders: A Meta-Analysis of Randomized Placebo-Controlled Trials," *Depression and Anxiety* 35, no. 6 (2018): 502–14.

6. Andrews, G., et al., "Royal Australian and New Zealand College of Psychiatrists Clinical Practice Guidelines for the Treatment of Panic Disorder, Social Anxiety Disorder and Generalised Anxiety Disorder," *Australian & New Zealand Journal of Psychiatry* 52, no. 12 (2018): 1109–72.

Bouchard, S., et al., "Virtual Reality Compared with In Vivo Exposure in the Treatment of Social Anxiety Disorder: A Three-Arm Randomised Controlled Trial," *The British Journal of Psychiatry* 210, no. 4 (2017): 276–83.

7. Scaini et al., op. cit.

8. Penninx, B., et al., "Anxiety Disorders," *Lancet* 397, no. 10277 (2021): 914–27.

9. Rapee, R. M., and R. G. Heimberg, "A Cognitive-Behavioral Model of Anxiety in Social Phobia," *Behaviour Research and Therapy* 35, no. 8 (1997): 741–56.

Kaczkurkin, A. N., and E. B. Foa, "Cognitive-Behavioral Therapy for Anxiety Disorders: An Update on the Empirical Evidence," *Dialogues in Clinical Neuroscience* 17, no. 3 (2015): 337–46.

10. Andrews et al., op. cit.

11. Gosmann, N. P. et al., "Selective Serotonin Reuptake Inhibitors, and Serotonin and Norepinephrine Reuptake Inhibitors for Anxiety, Obsessive-Compulsive, and Stress Disorders: A 3-Level Network Meta-Analysis," *PLoS Medicine* 18, no. 6 (2021): e1003664.

Mayo-Wilson, E., et al., "Psychological and Pharmacological Interventions for Social Anxiety Disorder in Adults: A Systematic Review and Network Meta-Analysis," *The Lancet Psychiatry* 1, no. 5 (2014): 368–76.

12. Andrews et al., op. cit.

Mitsui, N., et al., "Antidepressants for Social Anxiety Disorder: A Systematic Review and Meta-Analysis," *Neuropsychopharmacology Reports* 42, no. 4 (2022): 398–409.

13. Bernstein, D. A., et al., *New Directions in Progressive Relaxation Training: A Guidebook for Helping Professionals* (Westport: Praeger Publishers/Greenwood Publishing Group, Inc., 2000).

14. Szuhany, K. L., and N. M. Simon, "Anxiety Disorders: A Review," *JAMA* 328, no. 24 (2022): 2431–45.

15. Alomari, N., et al., "Social Anxiety Disorder: Associated Conditions and Therapeutic Approaches," *Cureus* 14, no. 12 (2022): e32687.

5. Panic Disorder

1. Batelaan, N. M., et al., "Panic Attacks as a Dimension of Psychopathology: Evidence for Associations with Onset and Course of Mental Disorders and Level of Functioning," *The Journal of Clinical Psychiatry* 73, no. 9 (2012): 1195–202.

2. Chang, H.-M., et al., "Identification and Medical Utilization of Newly Diagnosed Panic Disorder: A Nationwide Case–Control Study," *Journal of Psychosomatic Research* 125 (2019): 109815.

Fleet, R., et al., "Is Panic Disorder Associated with Coronary Artery Disease? A Critical Review of the Literature," *Journal of Psychosomatic Research* 48, no. 4–5 (2000): 347–56.

3. Pergamin-Hight, L., et al., "Content Specificity of Attention Bias to Threat in Anxiety Disorders: A Meta-Analysis," *Clinical Psychology Review* 35 (2015): 10–18.

4. American Psychiatric Association, *Diagnostic and Statistical Manual of Mental Disorders, Fifth Edition, Text Revision* (Washington, DC: American Psychiatric Association Publishing, 2022).

5. Remes, O., et al., "A Systematic Review of Reviews on the Prevalence of Anxiety Disorders in Adult Populations," *Brain and Behavior* 6, no. 7 (2016): e00497.

Kessler, R. C., et al., "Lifetime Prevalence and Age-of-Onset Distributions of DSM-IV Disorders in the National Comorbidity Survey Replication," *Archives of General Psychiatry* 62, no. 6 (2005): 593–602.

6. Andrews, G., et al., "Royal Australian and New Zealand College of Psychiatrists Clinical Practice Guidelines for the Treatment of Panic Disorder, Social Anxiety Disorder and Generalised Anxiety Disorder," *Australian & New Zealand Journal of Psychiatry* 52, no. 12 (2018): 1109–72.

Cuijpers, P., et al., "Relative Effects of Cognitive and Behavioral Therapies on Generalized Anxiety Disorder, Social Anxiety Disorder and Panic Disorder: A Meta-Analysis," *Journal of Anxiety Disorders* 43 (2016): 79–89.

"Generalised Anxiety Disorder and Panic Disorder in Adults: Management," National Institute for Health and Care Excellence, June 15, 2020, nice.org.uk/guidance/cg113/resources/generalised-anxiety-disorder-and-panic-disorder-in-adults-management-pdf-35109387756997.

7. Papola, D., et al., "CBT Treatment Delivery Formats for Panic Disorder: A Systematic Review and Network Meta-Analysis of Randomised Controlled Trials," *Psychological Medicine* 53, no. 3 (2023): 614–24.

8. Clark, D. M., "A Cognitive Model of Panic Attacks," in S. Rachman and J. D. Maser (eds.), *Panic: Psychological Perspectives* (Hillsdale: Erlbaum, 1988), 71–89.

9. Kyriakoulis, P., and M. Kyrios, "Biological and Cognitive Theories Explaining Panic Disorder: A Narrative Review," *Frontiers in Psychiatry* 14 (2023): 957515.

10. Kaczkurkin, A. N., and E. B. Foa, "Cognitive-Behavioral Therapy for Anxiety Disorders: An Update on the Empirical Evidence," *Dialogues in Clinical Neuroscience* 17, no. 3 (2015): 337–46.

11. Cuijpers et al., op. cit.

12. Ziffra, M., "Panic Disorder: A Review of Treatment Options," *Annals of Clinical Psychiatry* 33, no. 2 (2021): 124–33.

13. Chawla, N., et al., "Drug Treatment for Panic Disorder with or without Agoraphobia: Systematic Review and Network Meta-Analysis of Randomised Controlled Trials," *BMJ* 376 (2022): e066084.

14. "Generalised Anxiety Disorder and Panic Disorder," op. cit.

Dodds, T. J., "Prescribed Benzodiazepines and Suicide Risk: A Review of the Literature," *The Primary Care Companion for CNS Disorders* 19, no. 2 (2017): 22746.

Parsaik, A. K., et al., "Mortality Associated with Anxiolytic and Hypnotic Drugs: A Systematic Review and Meta-Analysis," *Australian and New Zealand Journal of Psychiatry* 50, no. 6 (2016): 520–33.

15. Bourin, M., et al., "Neurobiology of Panic Disorder," *Journal of Psychosomatic Research* 44, no. 1 (1998): 163–80.

16. Berkowitz, R. L., et al., "The Human Dimension: How the Prefrontal Cortex Modulates the Subcortical Fear Response," *Reviews in the Neurosciences* 18, no. 3–4 (2007): 191–207.

Schenberg, L. C., "Towards a Translational Model of Panic Attack," *Psychology & Neuroscience* 3, no. 1 (2010): 9–37.

17. Fleet et al., op. cit.

18. Batelaan et al., op. cit.

19. Lamers, F., et al., "Comorbidity Patterns of Anxiety and Depressive Disorders in a Large Cohort Study: The Netherlands Study of Depression and Anxiety (NESDA)," *The Journal of Clinical Psychiatry* 72, no. 3 (2011): 341–48.

20. Baker, H. J., et al., "Adolescents' Lived Experience of Panic Disorder: An Interpretative Phenomenological Analysis," *BMC Psychology* 10, no. 1 (2022): 143.

21. Ibid.

6. Trauma and Post-Traumatic Stress Disorder

1. Sherin, J. E., and C. B. Nemeroff, "Post-Traumatic Stress Disorder: The Neurobiological Impact of Psychological Trauma," *Dialogues in Clinical Neuroscience* 13, no. 3 (2011): 263–78.

2. Yehuda, R., et al., "Post-Traumatic Stress Disorder," *Nature Reviews Disease Primers* 1 (2015): 15057.

3. Bryant, R. A., "Post-Traumatic Stress Disorder: A State-of-the-Art Review of Evidence and Challenges," *World Psychiatry: Official Journal of the World Psychiatric Association (WPA)* 18, no. 3 (2019): 259–69.

4. American Psychiatric Association, *Diagnostic and Statistical Manual of Mental Disorders, Fifth Edition, Text Revision* (Washington, DC: American Psychiatric Association Publishing, 2022).

5. Lewis, C., et al., "Psychological Therapies for Post-Traumatic Stress Disorder in Adults: Systematic Review and Meta-Analysis," *European Journal of Psychotraumatology* 11, no. 1 (2020): 1729633.

6. De Jongh, A., et al., "Critical Analysis of The Current Treatment Guidelines for Complex PTSD in Adults," *Depression and Anxiety* 33, no. 5 (2016): 359–369. doi:10.1002/da.22469.

7. Deblinger, E., et al., "Disseminating Trauma-Focused Cognitive Behavioral Therapy with a Systematic Self-care Approach to Addressing Secondary Traumatic Stress: PRACTICE What You Preach," *Community Mental Health Journal* 56 (2020): 1531–43.

8. Anderson, F. G., *Transcending Trauma: Healing Complex PTSD with Internal Family Systems Therapy* (Eau Claire, WI: PESI Publishing, Inc., 2021).

9. Zaccari, B., et al., "Findings from a pilot study of Trauma Center Trauma-Sensitive Yoga versus cognitive processing therapy for PTSD related to military sexual trauma among women Veterans," *Complementary Therapies in Medicine* 70 (2022): 102850.

10. Williams, T., et al., "Pharmacotherapy for Post-Traumatic Stress Disorder (PTSD)," *Cochrane Database of Systematic Reviews* 3, no. 3 (2022): CD002795.

11. Panneton, W. M., and Q. Gan, "The Mammalian Diving Response: Inroads to Its Neural Control," *Frontiers in Neuroscience* 14 (2020): 524.

12. Siegel, D. J., *The Developing Mind: How Relationships and the Brain Interact to Shape Who We Are* (New York: Guilford Press, 2015).

13. Bryant, op. cit.

14. Twombly, J., *Trauma and Dissociation Informed Internal Family Systems: How to Successfully Treat C-PTSD, and Dissociative Disorders* (self-published, 2022).

15. *Mobbs, D., et al., "The Ecology of Human Fear: Survival Optimization and the Nervous System,"* Frontiers in Neuroscience *9 (2015): 55.*

16. Farrell, T., *"Window of Tolerance Reimagined,"* YouTube video, posted July 6, 2018, youtu.be/ZVEDueyZ2C4.

7. Developmental Trauma

1. Felitti, V. J., et al., "Relationship of Childhood Abuse and Household Dysfunction to Many of the Leading Causes of Death in Adults: The Adverse Childhood Experiences (ACE) Study," *American Journal of Preventive Medicine* 14, no. 4 (1998): 245–58.

2. World Health Organization, *International Statistical Classification of Diseases and Related Health Problems*, 11th edition (2019).

3. Felitti et al., op. cit.

4. Children's Defense Fund, "The State of America's Children 2023: Child Poverty," July 20, 2023, childrensdefense.org/tools-and-resources/the-state-of-americas-children/soac-child-poverty.

5. Chappell, K. K., et al., "Can We Ask Everyone? Addressing Sexual Abuse in Primary Care," *The Journal for Nurse Practitioners* 17, no. 5 (2021): 594–99.

6. Mainali, P., et al., "From Child Abuse to Developing Borderline Personality Disorder into Adulthood: Exploring the Neuromorphological and Epigenetic Pathway," *Cureus* 12, no. 7 (2020): e9474.

7. Harden, B. J., et al., "Maltreatment in Infancy: A Developmental Perspective on Prevention and Intervention," *Trauma, Violence, & Abuse* 17, no. 4 (2016): 366–86.

8. "Child Sexual Abuse Statistics," National Center for Victims of Crime, victimsofcrime.org/child-sexual-abuse-statistics. Accessed May 7, 2024.

9. Scoglio, A., et al., "Systematic Review of Risk and Protective Factors for Revictimization After Child Sexual Abuse," *Trauma, Violence & Abuse* 22, no. 1 (2021): 41–53.

10. Ibid.

11. Berger, E., et al., "Early Childhood Professionals' Perspectives on Dealing with Trauma of Children," *School Mental Health* 15, no. 1 (2023): 300–11.

12. Mainali et al., op. cit.

13. Wolynn, M., *It Didn't Start With You: How Inherited Family Trauma Shapes Who We Are and How to End the Cycle* (New York: Penguin, 2016).

14. Siegel, D. J., and M. Hartzell, *Parenting from the Inside Out: How a Deeper Self-Understanding Can Help You Raise Children Who Thrive* (New York: TarcherPerigee, 2013).

15. Scoglio, A. A. J., et al., "Self-Compassion and Responses to Trauma: The Role of Emotion Regulation," *Journal of Interpersonal Violence* 33, no. 13 (2018): 2016–36.

16. Chappell et al., op. cit.

Berger et al., op. cit.

17. Ringenberg, T. R., et al., "A Scoping Review of Child Grooming Strategies: Pre- and Post-Internet," *Child Abuse & Neglect* 123 (2022): 105392.

18. Feldman, R., "What Is Resilience: An Affiliative Neuroscience Approach," *World Psychiatry: Official Journal of the World Psychiatric Association (WPA)* 19, no. 2 (2020): 132–50.

19. Harden et al., op. cit.

20. Herringa, R. J., "Trauma, PTSD, and the Developing Brain," *Current Psychiatry Reports* 19, no. 10 (2017): 69.

21. "Missed Opportunities: LGBTQ Youth Homelessness in America," Chapin Hall at the University of Chicago, chapinhall.org/wp-content/uploads/VoYC-LGBTQ-Brief-FINAL.pdf. Accessed May 7, 2024.

22. Melegkovits, E., et al., "The Effectiveness of Trauma-Focused Psychotherapy for Complex Post-Traumatic Stress Disorder: A Retrospective Study," *European Psychiatry: The Journal of the Association of European Psychiatrists* 66, no. 1 (2022): e4.

23. Scoglio et al., op. cit.

8. Borderline Personality Disorder

1. Klein, P., et al., "Structural Stigma and Its Impact on Healthcare for Borderline Personality Disorder: A Scoping Review," *International Journal of Mental Health Systems* 16 (2022): 48.

2. Mainali, P., et al., "From Child Abuse to Developing Borderline Personality Disorder into Adulthood: Exploring the Neuromorphological and Epigenetic Pathway," *Cureus* 12, no. 7 (2020): e9474.

3. Carey, B., "Expert on Mental Illness Reveals Her Own Fight," *The New York Times*, June 23, 2011.

4. Klein et al., op. cit.

5. Ibid.

6. Price, D., *Unmasking Autism: Discovering the New Faces of Neurodiversity* (New York: Penguin Random House, 2022).

7. Gillespie, C., et al., "Dialectical Behavior Therapy for Individuals With Borderline Personality Disorder: A Systematic Review of Outcomes After One Year of Follow-Up," *Journal of Personality Disorders* 36, no. 4 (2022): 431–54.

8. Mainali, et al., op. cit.

9. Hepp, J., et al., "Linking Daily-Life Interpersonal Stressors and Health Problems Via Affective Reactivity in Borderline Personality and Depressive Disorders," *Psychosomatic Medicine* 82, no. 1 (2020): 90–98.

10. Fineberg, S. K., et al., "A Pilot Randomized Controlled Trial of Ketamine in Borderline Personality Disorder," *Neuropsychopharmacology* 48, no. 7 (2023): 991–99.

11. Perrotta, G., "Borderline Personality Disorder: Definition, Differential Diagnosis, Clinical Contexts, and Therapeutic Approaches," *Annals of Psychiatry and Treatment* 4, no. 1 (2020): 43–56.

12. Ibid.

13. Knaak, S., et al., "Stigma towards Borderline Personality Disorder: Effectiveness and Generalizability of an Anti-stigma Program for Healthcare Providers Using a Pre-post Randomized Design," *Borderline Personality Disorder and Emotion Dysregulation* 2 (2015): 9.

14. Mendez-Miller, M., et al., "Borderline Personality Disorder," *American Family Physician* 105, no. 2 (2022): 156–61.

15. Klein et al., op. cit.

16. Vanwoerden, S., et al., "The Relations between Inadequate Parent-Child Boundaries and Borderline Personality Disorder in Adolescence," *Psychiatry Research* 257 (2017): 462–71.

9. Attention-Deficit/Hyperactivity Disorder

1. Cundari, M., et al., "Neurocognitive and Cerebellar Function in ADHD, Autism and Spinocerebellar Ataxia," *Frontiers in Systems Neuroscience* 17 (2023): 1168666.

Dorr, M. M., and K. J. Armstrong, "Executive Functioning and Impairment in Emerging Adult College Students with ADHD Symptoms," *Journal of Attention Disorders* 23, no. 14 (2019): 1759–65.

Soto, E. F., et al., "Executive Functions and Writing Skills in Children With and Without ADHD," *Neuropsychology* 35, no. 8 (2021): 792–808.

2. LeFevre-Levy, R., et al., "Neurodiversity in the Workplace: Considering Neuroatypicality as a Form of Diversity," *Industrial and Organizational Psychology* 16, no. 1 (2023): 1–19.

3. Ibid.

Ananth, M., et al., "Dopamine D4 Receptor Gene Expression Plays Important Role in Extinction and Reinstatement of Cocaine-Seeking Behavior in Mice," *Behavioural Brain Research* 365 (2019): 1–6.

4. American Psychiatric Association, *Diagnostic and Statistical Manual of Mental Disorders, Fifth Edition, Text Revision* (Washington, DC: American Psychiatric Association Publishing, 2022).

5. Ahlberg, R., et al., "Real-Life Instability in ADHD from Young to Middle Adulthood: A Nationwide Register-Based Study of Social and Occupational Problems," *BMC Psychiatry* 23 (2023): 336.

6. Holbrook, J. R., et al., "Persistence of Parent-Reported ADHD Symptoms from Childhood Through Adolescence in a Community Sample," *Journal of Attention Disorders* 20, no. 1 (2016): 11–20.

7. Agnew-Blais, J. C., et al., "Persistence, Remission and Emergence of ADHD in Young Adulthood: Results from a Longitudinal, Prospective Population-Based Cohort," *JAMA Psychiatry* 73, no. 7 (2016): 713–20.

8. Quinn, P. O., and M. Madhoo, "A Review of Attention-Deficit/Hyperactivity Disorder in Women and Girls: Uncovering This Hidden Diagnosis," *The Primary Care Companion for CNS Disorders* 16, no. 3 (2014).

9. Faraone, S. V., et al., "The World Federation of ADHD International Consensus Statement: 208 Evidence-Based Conclusions About the Disorder," *Neuroscience & Biobehavioral Reviews* 128 (2021): 789–818.

10. Kazda, L., et al., "Overdiagnosis of Attention-Deficit/Hyperactivity Disorder in Children and Adolescents: A Systematic Scoping Review," *JAMA Network Open* 4, no. 4 (2021): e215335.

11. Faraone et al., op. cit.

Pastor, P., et al., "Association between Diagnosed ADHD and Selected Characteristics among Children Aged 4–17 Years: United States, 2011–2013," *NCHS Data Brief* no. 201 (2015).

Wetterer, L., "Attention-Deficit/Hyperactivity Disorder: AAP Updates Guideline for Diagnosis and Management," *American Family Physician* 102, no. 1 (2020): 58–60.

12. Quinn and Madhoo, op. cit.

13. Caye, A., et al., "Treatment Strategies for ADHD: An Evidence-Based Guide to Select Optimal Treatment," *Molecular Psychiatry* 24, no. 3 (2019): 390–408.

14. Boland, H., et al., "A Literature Review and Meta-Analysis on the Effects of ADHD Medications on Functional Outcomes," *Journal of Psychiatric Research* 123 (2020): 21–30.

15. Faraone et al., op. cit.

Wetterer, op. cit.

Wolraich, Mark L. et al., "Clinical Practice Guideline for the Diagnosis, Evaluation, and Treatment of Attention-Deficit/Hyperactivity Disorder in Children and Adolescents," *Pediatrics* 144, no. 4 (2019): e20192528.

16. Deang, K. T., et al., "The Novelty of Bupropion as a Dopaminergic Antidepressant for the Treatment of Adult Attention Deficit Hyperactive Disorder," *Current Drug Targets* 20, no. 2 (2019): 210–19.

17. Faraone et al., op. cit.

Fullen, T., et al., "Psychological Treatments in Adult ADHD: A Systematic Review," *Journal of Psychopathology and Behavioral Assessment* 42 (2020): 500–18.

Knouse, L. E., et al., "Meta-Analysis of Cognitive–Behavioral Treatments for Adult ADHD," *Journal of Consulting and Clinical Psychology* 85, no. 7 (2017): 737–50.

Lopez, P. L., et al., "Cognitive-behavioural interventions for attention deficit hyperactivity disorder (ADHD) in adults," *Cochrane Database of Systematic Reviews* 3, no. 3 (2018): CD010840.

18. Knouse et al., op. cit.

19. Wolraich et al., op. cit.

20. Morrow, R. L., et al., "Influence of Relative Age on Diagnosis and Treatment of Attention-Deficit/Hyperactivity Disorder in Children," *CMAJ: Canadian Medical Association Journal* 184, no. 7 (2012): 755–62.

21. Boland et al., op. cit.

Wolraich et al., op. cit.

22. Cundari et al., op. cit.

Faraone et al., op. cit.

23. Cundari et al., op. cit.

Stoodley, C. J., "The Cerebellum and Neurodevelopmental Disorders," *Cerebellum* 15, no. 1 (2016): 34–37.

24. Mehta, T. R., et al., "Neurobiology of ADHD: A Review," *Current Developmental Disorders Reports* 6, no. 4 (2019): 235–40.

25. Faraone et al., op. cit.

26. van der Voet, M., et al., "ADHD-associated dopamine transporter, latrophilin and neurofibromin share a dopamine-related locomotor signature in Drosophila," *Molecular Psychiatry* 21, no. 4 (2016): 565–73.

27. Becker, S. P., "ADHD and Sleep: Recent Advances and Future Directions," *Current Opinion in Psychology* 34 (2020): 50–56.

28. Singh, K., and A. W. Zimmerman, "Sleep in Autism Spectrum Disorder and Attention Deficit Hyperactivity Disorder," *Seminars in Pediatric Neurology* 22, no. 2 (2015): 113–25.

29. Wilson, D. E., *The Polyvagal Path to Joyful Learning: Transforming Classrooms One Nervous System at a Time* (New York: W. W. Norton, 2023).

30. Bornstein, M. H., and G. Esposito, "Coregulation: A Multilevel Approach via Biology and Behavior," *Children* 10, no. 8 (2023): 1323.

31. Cibrian, F. L., et al., "The Potential for Emerging Technologies to Support Self-Regulation in Children with ADHD: A Literature Review," *International Journal of Child-Computer Interaction* 31 (2021): 100421.

32. Lambez, B., et al., "Non-Pharmacological Interventions for Cognitive Difficulties in ADHD: A Systematic Review and Meta-Analysis," *Journal of Psychiatric Research* 120 (2020): 40–55.

33. Boland et al., op. cit.

Wolraich et al., op. cit.

34. American Psychiatric Association, op. cit.

Dwyer, P., "The Neurodiversity Approach(es): What Are They and What Do They Mean for Researchers?," *Human Development* 66, no. 2 (2022): 73–92.

35. American Psychiatric Association, op. cit.

36. Mark, T. L., et al., "Differential Reimbursement of Psychiatric Services by Psychiatrists and Other Medical Providers," *Psychiatric Services* 69, no. 3 (2018): 281–85.

Pelech, D., and T. Hayford, "Medicare Advantage and Commercial Prices for Mental Health Services," *Health Affairs* 38, no. 2 (2019): 262–67.

37. Kazda, L., et al., "Association of Attention-Deficit/Hyperactivity Disorder Diagnosis with Adolescent Quality of Life," *JAMA Network Open* 5, no. 10 (2022): e2236364.

38. Agnew-Blais et al., op. cit.

39. Wolraich et al., op. cit.

Centers for Disease Control and Prevention, "Mental Health in the United States: Prevalence of Diagnosis and Medication Treatment for Attention-Deficit/Hyperactivity Disorder—United States, 2003," *MMWR Morbidity and Mortality Weekly Report* 54, no. 34 (2005): 842–47.

40. Faraone et al., op. cit.

41. National Collaborating Centre for Mental Health, *Attention Deficit Hyperactivity Disorder: Diagnosis and Management of ADHD in Children, Young People and Adults* (Leicester: British Psychological Society, 2009).

10. Interpersonal Relationships

1. Bacon, I., et al., "The Lived Experience of Codependency: An Interpretative Phenomenological Analysis," *International Journal of Mental Health and Addiction* 18 (2020): 754–771.

2. Johnson, B. T., and R. L. Acabchuk, "What Are the Keys to a Longer, Happier Life? Answers from Five Decades of Health Psychology Research," *Social Science & Medicine* 196 (2018): 218–26.

3. Beasley, C. C., and R. Ager, "Emotionally Focused Couples Therapy: A Systematic Review of Its Effectiveness over the Past 19 Years," *Journal of Evidence-Based Social Work* 16, no. 2 (2019): 144–59.

Greenberg, L. S., and S. M. Johnson, *Emotionally Focused Therapy for Couples* (New York: Guilford Press, 1988).

4. Diamond, G., et al., "Attachment-Based Family Therapy: A Review of the Empirical Support," *Family Process* 55, no. 3 (2016): 595–610.

5. Grewen, K. M., et al., "Warm Partner Contact Is Related to Lower Cardiovascular Reactivity," *Behavioral Medicine* 29, no. 3 (2003): 123–30.

6. Prochaska, J. O., and C. C. DiClemente, "Stages and processes of self-change of smoking: toward an integrative model of change," *Journal of Consulting and Clinical Psychology* 51, no. 3 (1983): 390.

7. Raihan, N., and M. Cogburn., "Stages of Change Theory," in: StatPearls, (Treasure Island: StatPearls Publishing; 2023). ncbi.nlm.nih.gov/books/NBK556005/.

8. Shaffer, J. A., "Stages-of-Change Model," in M. D. Gellman and J. R. Turner (eds.), *Encyclopedia of Behavioral Medicine* (New York: Springer, 2013).

9. "The Loneliness Epidemic Persists: A Post-Pandemic Look at the State of Loneliness Among US Adults," The Cigna Group, May 26, 2022, newsroom.thecignagroup.com/loneliness-epidemic-persists-post-pandemic-look.

10. Office of the Surgeon General, "Our Epidemic of Loneliness and Isolation: The US Surgeon General's Advisory on the Healing Effects of Social Connection and Community" (Washington, DC: US Department of Health and Human Services, 2023).

11. Loneliness

1. Holt-Lunstad, J., et al., "Advancing Social Connection as a Public Health Priority in the United States," *American Psychologist* 72, no. 6 (2017): 517–30.

2. Perlman, D., and L. A. Peplau, "Toward a Social Psychology of Loneliness," in R. Gilmour and S. Duck (eds.), *Personal Relationships: 3. Relationships in Disorder* (London: Academic Press, 1981), 31–56.

3. Holt-Lunstad, J., et al., "Loneliness and Social Isolation as Risk Factors for Mortality: A Meta-Analytic Review," *Perspectives on Psychological Science* 10, no. 2 (2015): 227–37.

4. Ibid.

Bruce, L. D. H., et al., "Loneliness in the United States: A 2018 National Panel Survey of Demographic, Structural, Cognitive, and Behavioral Characteristics," *American Journal of Health Promotion* 33, no. 8 (2019): 1123–33.

5. Office of the Surgeon General, "Our Epidemic of Loneliness and Isolation: The US Surgeon General's Advisory on the Healing Effects of Social Connection and Community" (Washington, DC: US Department of Health and Human Services, 2023).

Surkalim, D. L., et al., "The Prevalence of Loneliness across 113 Countries: Systematic Review and Meta-Analysis," *BMJ* 376 (2022): e067068.

6. "The Loneliness Epidemic Persists: A Post-Pandemic Look at the State of Loneliness Among US Adults," The Cigna Group, May 26, 2022, newsroom.thecignagroup.com/loneliness-epidemic-persists-post-pandemic-look.

7. Heng, S., *Let's Talk About Loneliness: The Search for Connection in a Lonely World* (London: Hay House, 2023).

8. Yanguas, J., S., et al., "The Complexity of Loneliness," *Acta Biomedica* 89, no. 2 (2018): 302–14.

9. Goossens, L., et al., "The Genetics of Loneliness: Linking Evolutionary Theory to Genome-Wide Genetics, Epigenetics, and Social Science," *Perspectives on Psychological Science* 10, no. 2 (2015): 213–26.

10. Auyeung, B., et al., "Oxytocin Increases Eye Contact during a Real-Time, Naturalistic Social Interaction in Males with and without Autism," *Translational Psychiatry* 5, no. 2 (2015): e507.

Prinsen, J., et al., "To Mirror or Not to Mirror upon Mutual Gaze, Oxytocin Can Pave the Way: A Cross-over Randomized Placebo-Controlled Trial," *Psychoneuroendocrinology* 90 (2018): 148–56.

11. O'Day, E. B., and R. G. Heimberg, "Social Media Use, Social Anxiety, and Loneliness: A Systematic Review," *Computers in Human Behavior Reports* 3 (2021): 100070.

12. Seabrook, E. M., et al., "Social Networking Sites, Depression, and Anxiety: A Systematic Review," *JMIR Mental Health* 3, no. 4 (2016): e50.

13. O'Day and Heimberg, op. cit.

14. Seabrook et al., op. cit.

15. Hunt, M. G., et al., "No More FOMO: Limiting Social Media Decreases Loneliness and Depression," *Journal of Social and Clinical Psychology* 37, no. 10 (2018): 751–68.

16. Heng, op. cit.

17. Beutel, M. E., et al., "Loneliness in the General Population: Prevalence, Determinants and Relations to Mental Health," *BMC Psychiatry* 17, no. 1 (2017).

Erzen, E., and Ö. Çikrikci, "The Effect of Loneliness on Depression: A Meta-Analysis," *International Journal of Social Psychiatry* 64, no. 5 (2018): 427–35.

18. Bruce et al., "Loneliness in the United States," 1123–33.

19. Valtorta, N. K., et al., "Loneliness and Social Isolation as Risk Factors for Coronary Heart Disease and Stroke: Systematic Review and Meta-Analysis of Longitudinal Observational Studies," *Heart* 102, no. 13 (2016): 1009–16.

12. Work Stress and Burnout

1. "Mental Health at Work: Managers and Money," The Workforce Institute at UKG, 2023, ukg.com/sites/default/files/2023-01/CV2040-Part2-UKG%20Global%20Survey%202023-Manager%20Impact%20on%20Mental%20Health-Final.pdf.

2. "Occupational Health: Stress at the Workplace," World Health Organization, October 19, who.int/news-room/questions-and-answers/item/ccupational-health-stress-at-the-workplace.

3. "Burnout," ICD-11 for Mortality and Morbidity Statistics, World Health Organization, icd.who.int/browse/2024-01/mms/en#129180281. Accessed May 7, 2024.

4. Goh, J., et al., "The Relationship between Workplace Stressors and Mortality and Health Costs in the United States," *Management Science* 62, no. 2 (2016): 608–28.

5. "Workplace Stress," Occupational Safety and Health Administration, osha.gov/workplace-stress/understanding-the-problem. Accessed May 7, 2024.

6. "Mental Health at Work," op. cit.

7. Ibid.

8. Clark, P., et al., "The Impostor Phenomenon in Mental Health Professionals: Relationships among Compassion Fatigue, Burnout, and Compassion Satisfaction," *Contemporary Family Therapy* 44, no. 2 (2022): 185–97.

9. Bravata, D. M., et al., "Prevalence, Predictors, and Treatment of Impostor Syndrome: A Systematic Review," *Journal of General Internal Medicine* 35, no. 4 (2020): 1252–75.

10. Koutsimani, P., et al., "The Relationship between Burnout, Depression, and Anxiety: A Systematic Review and Meta-Analysis," *Frontiers in Psychology* 10 (2019): 284.

13. Grief

1. O'Connor, M.-F., "Grief: A Brief History of Research on How Body, Mind, and Brain Adapt," *Psychosomatic Medicine* 81, no. 8 (2019): 731–38.

2. O'Connor, M.-F., *The Grieving Brain: The Surprising Science of How We Learn from Love and Loss* (San Francisco: HarperOne, 2022).

3. American Psychiatric Association, *Diagnostic and Statistical Manual of Mental Disorders, Fifth Edition, Text Revision* (Washington, DC: American Psychiatric Association Publishing, 2022).

4. Breen, L. J., et al., "A Co-Designed Systematic Review and Meta-Analysis of the Efficacy of Grief Interventions for Anxiety and Depression in Young People," *Journal of Affective Disorders* 335 (2023): 289–97.

Szuhany, K. L., et al., "Prolonged Grief Disorder: Course, Diagnosis, Assessment, and Treatment," *Focus* 19, no. 2 (2021): 161–72.

5. Ibid.

6. Helbert, K., *Yoga for Grief and Loss: Poses, Meditation, Devotion, Self-Reflection, Selfless Acts, Ritual* (Philadelphia: Singing Dragon, 2015).

O'Shea, M., et al., "Integration of Hatha Yoga and Evidence-Based Psychological Treatments for Common Mental Disorders: An Evidence Map," *Journal of Clinical Psychology* 78, no. 9 (2022): 1671–711.

Sausys, A., *Yoga for Grief Relief: Simple Practices for Transforming Your Grieving Mind and Body* (Oakland: New Harbinger Publications, 2014).

7. Shulman, L., "Healing Your Brain After Loss: A Neurologist's Perspective," American Brain Foundation, June 24, 2021, youtube.com/watch?v=hZwhslOz7qY.

8. Bonanno, G. A., *The Other Side of Sadness: What the New Science of Bereavement Tells Us about Life after Loss* (London: Hachette UK, 2019).

14. Infertility and Pregnancy Loss

1. Belluck, P., "Use of Abortion Pills Rose Significantly Post Roe, Research Shows," The New York Times, March 25, 2024.

2. "Infertility," Centers for Disease Control and Prevention, cdc.gov/reproductivehealth/infertility/index.htm. Accessed May 7, 2024.

3. Strumpf, E., et al., "Prevalence and Clinical, Social, and Health Care Predictors of Miscarriage," *BMC Pregnancy Childbirth* 21, no. 1 (2021): 185.

4. Agarwal, A., et al., "Male Infertility," *Lancet* 397, no. 10271 (2021): 319–33.

5. Osadchiy, V., et al., "Understanding Patient Anxieties in the Social Media Era: Qualitative Analysis and Natural Language Processing of an Online Male Infertility Community," *Journal of Medical Internet Research* 22, no. 3 (2020): e16728.

6. Zhou, R., et al., "Pregnancy or Psychological Outcomes of Psychotherapy Interventions for Infertility: A Meta-Analysis," *Frontiers in Psychology* 12 (2021): 643395.

7. Vučina, T., and S. Oakley, "Case Study of EMDR Therapy Use in Treating Reproductive Trauma—A Case Report," *Psychiatria Danubina* 30, suppl. 5 (2018): 262–64.

8. Gaitzsch, H., et al., "The Effect of Mind-Body Interventions on Psychological and Pregnancy Outcomes in Infertile Women: A Systematic Review," *Archives of Women's Mental Health* 23, no. 4 (2020): 479–91.

9. Kiani, Z., et al., "The Prevalence of Anxiety Symptoms in Infertile Women: A Systematic Review and Meta-Analysis," *Fertility Research and Practice* 6 (2020): 7.

10. Osadchiy et al., op. cit.

11. Tam, M. W., "Queering Reproductive Access: Reproductive Justice in Assisted Reproductive Technologies," *Reproductive Health* 18, no. 1 (2021): 164.

12. Lett, E., et al., "Community Support Persons and Mitigating Obstetric Racism During Childbirth," *Annals of Family Medicine* 21, no. 3 (2023): 227–33.

13. Tam, op. cit.

14. Kiani et al., op. cit.

Szkodziak, F., et al., "Psychological Aspects of Infertility: A Systematic Review," *The Journal of International Medical Research* 48, no. 6 (2020): 300060520932403.

15. Ibid.

15. Sexual Assault

1. Armstrong, E. A., et al., "Silence, Power, and Inequality: An Intersectional Approach to Sexual Violence," *Annual Review of Sociology* 44 (2018): 99–122.

2. "Criminal Justice System," Rape, Abuse, and Incest National Network, rainn.org/statistics/criminal-justice-system. Accessed May 7, 2024.

3. Cuevas, K. M., et al., "Neurobiology of Sexual Assault and Osteopathic Considerations for Trauma-Informed Care and Practice," *The Journal of the American Osteopathic Association* 118, no. 2 (2018): e2–10.

4. "Perpetrators of Sexual Violence," Rape, Abuse, and Incest National Network, rainn.org/statistics/perpetrators-sexual-violence. Accessed May 7, 2024.

5. Cuevas et al., op. cit.

6. Carli, G., and F. Farabollini, "Chapter 12—Tonic Immobility as a Survival, Adaptive Response and as a Recovery Mechanism," *Progress in Brain Research* 271, no. 1 (2022): 305–29.

7. Farahi, N., and M. McEachern, "Sexual Assault of Women," *American Family Physician* 103, no. 3 (2021): 168–76.

8. Kalaf, J., et al., "Sexual Trauma Is More Strongly Associated with Tonic Immobility Than Other Types of Trauma—A Population Based Study," *Journal of Affective Disorders* 215 (2017): 71–76.

9. Kalaf, J., et al., "Peritraumatic Tonic Immobility in a Large Representative Sample of the General Population: Association with Posttraumatic Stress Disorder and Female Gender," *Comprehensive Psychiatry* 60 (2015): 68–72.

10. Roberts, N. P., et al., "Early Psychological Intervention Following Recent Trauma: A Systematic Review and Meta-Analysis," *European Journal of Psychotraumatology* 10, no. 1 (2019): 1695486.

11. Bohus, M., et al., "Dialectical Behavior Therapy for Posttraumatic Stress Disorder (DBT-PTSD) Compared with Cognitive Processing Therapy (CPT) in Complex Presentations of PTSD in Women Survivors of Childhood Abuse: A Randomized Clinical Trial," *JAMA Psychiatry* 77, no. 12 (2020): 1235–45.

12. Cuevas et al., op. cit.

13. Palmieri, J., and J. L. Valentine, "Using Trauma-Informed Care to Address Sexual Assault and Intimate Partner Violence in Primary Care," *The Journal for Nurse Practitioners* 17, no. 1 (2021): 44–48.

14. Ibid.

15. "Perpetrators of Sexual Violence," op. cit.

16. Hendricks, P., and S. Seybold, "Unauthorized Pelvic Exams Are Sexual Assault," *The New Bioethics* 28, no. 4 (2022): 368–76.

17. Gómez-Durán, E. L., and C. Martin-Fumadó, "Nonconsensual Condom-Use Deception: An Empirically Based Conceptualization of Stealthing," *Trauma, Violence & Abuse* 25, no. 1 (2022): 87–101.

18. Palmieri and Valentine, op. cit.

19. Dworkin, E. R., "Risk for Mental Disorders Associated with Sexual Assault: A Meta-Analysis," *Trauma, Violence & Abuse* 21, no. 5 (2020): 1011–28.

20. de Aquino Ferreira, L. F., et al., "Borderline Personality Disorder and Sexual Abuse: A Systematic Review," *Psychiatry Research* 262 (2018): 70–77.

21. "Criminal Justice System," op. cit.

22. Barry, S., and E. Harris, "The Children's Programme: A Description of a Group and Family Intervention for Children Engaging in Problematic and Harmful Sexual Behaviour and Their Parents/Carers," *Journal of Sexual Aggression* 25, no. 2 (2019): 193–206.

23. Jenkins, C. S., et al., "Preliminary Findings of Problematic Sexual Behavior-Cognitive-Behavioral Therapy for Adolescents in an Outpatient Treatment Setting," *Child Abuse & Neglect* 105 (2020): 104428.

24. Kalaf et al., op. cit.

25. Cuevas et al., op. cit.

16. Intimate Partner Violence

1. "Understanding and Addressing Violence against Women: Intimate Partner Violence," World Health Organization and Pan American Health Organization, apps.who. int/iris/handle/10665/77432. Accessed May 7, 2024.

2. Sardinha, L., et al., "Global, Regional, and National Prevalence Estimates of Physical or Sexual, or Both, Intimate Partner Violence against Women in 2018," *The Lancet* 399, no. 10327 (2022): 803–13.

3. Sugg, N., "Intimate Partner Violence: Prevalence, Health Consequences, and Intervention," *Medical Clinics of North America* 99, no. 3 (2015): 629–49.

4. Sardinha et al., op. cit.

5. Sugg, op. cit.

6. Sweet, P. L., "The Sociology of Gaslighting," *American Sociological Review* 84, no. 5 (2019): 851–75.

7. Sugg, op. cit.

8. Liu, X., et al., "Cardiovascular Risk and Outcomes in Women Who Have Experienced Intimate Partner Violence: An Integrative Review," *Journal of Cardiovascular Nursing* 35, no. 4 (2020): 400–14.

9. MacMillan, H. L., and C. N. Wathen, "Children's Exposure to Intimate Partner Violence: Impacts and Interventions," *Child and Adolescent Psychiatric Clinics of North America* 23, no. 2 (2020): 295–308.

10. Cohen, J. A., et al., *Treating Trauma and Traumatic Grief in Children and Adolescents, Second Edition* (New York: Guilford Press, 2017).

17. Body Image

1. Voss, Patrice et al., "Dynamic Brains and the Changing Rules of Neuroplasticity: Implications for Learning and Recovery," *Frontiers in Psychology* 8 (2017): 1657.

2. Gattario, H., and A. Frisén, "From Negative to Positive Body Image: Men's and Women's Journeys from Early Adolescence to Emerging Adulthood," *Body Image* 28 (2019): 53–65.

3. Klimek, P., et al., "Cognitive Behavioral Therapy for Body Image and Self Care (CBT-BISC) among Sexual Minority Men Living with HIV: Skills-Based Treatment Mediators," *Cognitive Therapy and Research* 44, no. 1 (2020): 208–15.

4. He, J., et al., "Meta-analysis of Gender Differences in Body Appreciation," *Body Image* 33 (2020): 90–100.

5. Schimel, J., et al., "Not all Self-Affirmations Were Created Equal: The Cognitive and Social Benefits of Affirming the Intrinsic (Vs. Extrinsic) Self," *Social Cognition* 22, no. 1 (2004): 75–99.

6. Fioravanti, G., et al., "How the Exposure to Beauty Ideals on Social Networking Sites Influences Body Image: A Systematic Review of Experimental Studies," *Adolescent Research Review* 7 (2022): 419–58.

7. Gattario and Frisén, op. cit.

8. Ibid.

9. McGuire, J. K., et al., "Body Image in Transgender Young People: Findings from a Qualitative, Community Based Study," *Body Image* 18 (2016): 96–107.

10. Galupo, M. P., et al., "'Having a non-normative body for me is about survival': Androgynous Body Ideal among Trans and Nonbinary Individuals," *Body Image* 39 (2021): 68–76.

11. Tylka, T. L., and N. L. Wood-Barcalow, "What is and What is Not Positive Body Image? Conceptual Foundations and Construct Definition," *Body Image* 14 (2015): 118–29.

18. Relationship with Food

1. American Psychiatric Association, *Diagnostic and Statistical Manual of Mental Disorders, Fifth Edition, Text Revision* (Washington, DC: American Psychiatric Association Publishing, 2022).

2. Ibid.

3. Parker, L. L., and J. A. Harriger, "Eating Disorders and Disordered Eating Behaviors in the LGBT Population: A Review of the Literature," *Journal of Eating Disorders* 8 (2020): 51.

4. Brede, J., et al., "'For Me, the Anorexia Is Just a Symptom, and the Cause Is the Autism': Investigating Restrictive Eating Disorders in Autistic Women," *Journal of Autism and Developmental Disorders* 50, no. 12 (2020): 4280–96.

5. Kaisari, P., et al., "Associations between Core Symptoms of Attention Deficit Hyperactivity Disorder and Both Binge and Restrictive Eating," *Frontiers in Psychiatry* 9 (2018): 103.

6. Bourne, L., et al., "Avoidant/Restrictive Food Intake Disorder and Severe Food Selectivity in Children and Young People with Autism: A Scoping Review," *Developmental Medicine and Child Neurology* 64, no. 6 (2022): 691–700.

7. de Jong, M., et al., "Effectiveness of Enhanced Cognitive Behavior Therapy for Eating Disorders: A Randomized Controlled Trial," *International Journal of Eating Disorders* 53, no. 5 (2020): 717–27.

8. Steindl, S. R., et al., "Compassion Focused Therapy for Eating Disorders: A Qualitative Review and Recommendations for Further Applications," *Clinical Psychologist* 21, no. 2 (2017): 62–73.

9. Ibid.

10. Couturier, J., et al., "Canadian Practice Guidelines for the Treatment of Children and Adolescents with Eating Disorders," *Journal of Eating Disorders* 8 (2020): 4.

11. Tan, J. S. K., et al., "Eating Disorders in Children and Adolescents," *Singapore Medical Journal* 63, no. 6 (2022): 294–98.

12. Quesnel, D., et al., "Medical and Physiological Complications of Exercise for Individuals with an Eating Disorder: A Narrative Review," *Journal of Eating Disorders* 11, no. 1 (2023): 1–18.

13. Hambleton, A., et al., "Psychiatric and Medical Comorbidities of Eating Disorders: Findings from a Rapid Review of the Literature," *Journal of Eating Disorders* 10, no. 1 (2022): 132.

Mitchell, K. S., et al., "The Impact of Comorbid Posttraumatic Stress Disorder on Eating Disorder Treatment Outcomes: Investigating the Unified Treatment Model," *International Journal of Eating Disorders* 54, no. 7 (2021): 1260–69.

14. McCuen-Wurst, C., et al., "Weight and Eating Concerns in Women's Reproductive Health," *Current Psychiatry Reports* 19, no. 68 (2017): 1–10.

15. Tan et al., op. cit.

16. Ibid.

19. Addiction

1. Love Hardin, L., *The Many Lives of Mama Love: A Memoir of Lying, Stealing, Writing, and Healing* (New York: Simon & Schuster, 2023).

2. Rizk, M. M., et al., "Suicide Risk and Addiction: The Impact of Alcohol and Opioid Use Disorders," *Current Addiction Reports* 8, no. 2 (2021): 194–207.

3. American Psychiatric Association, *Diagnostic and Statistical Manual of Mental Disorders, Fifth Edition, Text Revision* (Washington, DC: American Psychiatric Association Publishing, 2022).

4. Ibid.

5. Ibid.

6. "Drug Misuse and Addiction," National Institute on Drug Abuse, nida.nih.gov/publications/drugs-brains-behavior-science-addiction/drug-misuse-addiction. Accessed May 7, 2024.

7. Markus, W., and H. K. Hornsveld, "EMDR Interventions in Addiction," *Journal of EMDR Practice and Research* 11, no. 1 (2017): 3–29.

8. American Psychiatric Association, *Diagnostic and Statistical Manual of Mental Disorders, Fifth Edition, Text Revision*, 2022.

9. Goh, C. M. J., et al., "Gender Differences in Alcohol Use: a Nationwide Study in a Multiethnic Population," *International Journal of Mental Health and Addiction* (2022).

10. "Key Substance Use and Mental Health Indicators in the United States: Results from the 2019 National Survey on Drug Use and Health," Substance Abuse and Mental Health Services Administration, samhsa.gov/data. Accessed May 7, 2024.

11. Dugosh, K., et al., "A Systematic Review on the Use of Psychosocial Interventions in Conjunction with Medications for the Treatment of Opioid Addiction," *Journal of Addiction Medicine* 10, no. 2 (2016): 91–101.

12. Marchand, K., et al., "Conceptualizing Patient-Centered Care for Substance Use Disorder Treatment: Findings from a Systematic Scoping Review," *Substance Abuse Treatment, Prevention, and Policy* 14, no. 1 (2019): 37.

13. Volkow, N. D., and M. Boyle, "Neuroscience of Addiction: Relevance to Prevention and Treatment," *American Journal of Psychiatry* 175, no. 8 (2018): 729–40.

14. Ibid.

15. "Treat Opioid Use Disorder," Centers for Disease Control and Prevention, National Center for Injury Prevention and Control, cdc.gov/opioids/overdoseprevention/treatment.html. Accessed May 7, 2024.

16. Volkow, N. D., "Personalizing the Treatment of Substance Use Disorders," *The American Journal of Psychiatry* 177, no. 2 (2020): 113–16.

17. Markus and Hornsveld, op. cit.

18. Tapia, G., "Review of EMDR Interventions for Individuals with Substance Use Disorder With/Without Comorbid Posttraumatic Stress Disorder," *Journal of EMDR Practice and Research* 13, no. 4 (2019): 345–53.

19. Ibid.

Markus and Hornsveld, op. cit.

20. Schindler, A., "Attachment and Substance Use Disorders—Theoretical Models, Empirical Evidence, and Implications for Treatment," *Frontiers in Psychiatry* 10 (2019): 727.

21. Kelly, J. F., et al., "Alcoholics Anonymous and 12-Step Facilitation Treatments for Alcohol Use Disorder: A Distillation of a 2020 Cochrane Review for Clinicians and Policy Makers," *Alcohol and Alcoholism* 55, no. 6 (2020): 641–51.

22. Volkow, op. cit.

23. Ibid.

24. "Key Substance Use and Mental Health Indicators," op. cit.

25. Interlandi, J., "48 Million Americans Live With Addiction. Here's How to Get Them Help That Works," *The New York Times*, December 13, 2023.

26. Rosenblatt, R. A., et al., "Geographic and Specialty Distribution of US Physicians Trained to Treat Opioid Use Disorder," *The Annals of Family Medicine* 13, no. 1 (2015): 23–26.

27. Samuels, E. A., et al., "Innovation During COVID-19: Improving Addiction Treatment Access," *Journal of Addiction Medicine* 14, no. 4 (2020): e8–9.

28. Olsen, Y., and J. M. Sharfstein, "Confronting the Stigma of Opioid Use Disorder—and Its Treatment," *JAMA* 311, no. 14 (2014): 1393–94.

29. Tsai, A. C., et al, "Stigma as a Fundamental Hindrance to the United States Opioid Overdose Crisis Response," *PLoS Medicine* 16, no. 11 (2019): e1002969.

Wakeman, S. E., and J. D. Rich, "Barriers to Medications for Addiction Treatment: How Stigma Kills," *Substance Use & Misuse* 53, no. 2 (2018): 330–33.

30. Volkow, op. cit.

31. Markus and Hornsveld, op. cit.

32. Eddie, D., et al., "Lived Experience in New Models of Care for Substance Use Disorder: A Systematic Review of Peer Recovery Support Services and Recovery Coaching," *Frontiers in Psychology* 10 (2019): 1052.

33. Yuodelis-Flores, C., and R. K. Ries, "Addiction and Suicide: A Review," *FOCUS, A Journal of the American Psychiatric Association* 17, no. 2 (2019): 193–99.

34. Ibid.

35. Brownlie, E., et al., "Early Adolescent Substance Use and Mental Health Problems and Service Utilisation in a School-based Sample," *The Canadian Journal of Psychiatry* 64, no. 2 (2019): 116–25.

36. Butelman, E. R., et al., "Age of Onset of Heaviest Use of Cannabis or Alcohol in Persons with Severe Opioid or Cocaine Use Disorders," *Drug and Alcohol Dependence* 226 (2021): 108834.

37. Otten, R., et al., "A Developmental Cascade Model for Early Adolescent-Onset Substance Use: The Role of Early Childhood Stress," *Addiction* 114, no. 2 (2019): 326–34.

20. Chronic Pain

1. Merskey, H., and N. Bogduk, *Classification of Chronic Pain*, 2nd edition (Seattle: IASP Press, 2011): 209–14.

2. Schwan, J., et al., "Chronic Pain Management in the Elderly," *Anesthesiology Clinics* 37, no. 3 (2019): 547–60.

3. Merskey and Bogduk, op.cit.

4. Clauw, D. J., et al., "Reframing Chronic Pain as a Disease, Not a Symptom: Rationale and Implications for Pain Management," *Postgraduate Medicine* 131, no. 3 (2019): 185–98.

5. Andrew, R., et al., "The Costs and Consequences of Adequately Managed Chronic Non-cancer Pain and Chronic Neuropathic Pain," *Pain Practice* 14, no. 1 (2014): 79–94.

6. Dueñas, M., et al., "A Review of Chronic Pain Impact on Patients, Their Social Environment and the Health Care System," *Journal of Pain Research* 28, no. 9 (2016): 457–67.

7. Schwan et al., op. cit.

Takai, Y., et al., "Literature Review of Pain Management for People with Chronic Pain," *Japan Journal of Nursing Science* 12, no. 3 (2015): 167–83.

8. Dale, R., and B. Stacey, "Multimodal Treatment of Chronic Pain," *Medical Clinics of North America* 100, no. 1 (2016): 55–64.

9. Clauw et al., op. cit.

Groenewald, C. B., et al., "Prevalence of Pain Management Techniques Among Adults with Chronic Pain in the United States, 2019," *JAMA Network Open* 5, no. 2 (2022): e2146697.

10. Andrew et al., op. cit.

Veehof, M. M., et al., "Acceptance- and Mindfulness-Based Interventions for the Treatment of Chronic Pain: A Meta-Analytic Review," *Cognitive Behaviour Therapy* 45, no. 1 (2016): 5–31.

11. Lin, I., et al., "What Does Best Practice Care for Musculoskeletal Pain Look Like? Eleven Consistent Recommendations from High-Quality Clinical Practice Guidelines: Systematic Review," *British Journal of Sports Medicine* 54, no. 2 (2020): 79–86.

12. Clauw et al., op. cit.

Ehde, D. M., et al., "Cognitive-Behavioral Therapy for Individuals with Chronic Pain: Efficacy, Innovations, and Directions for Research," *The American Psychologist* 69, no. 2 (2014): 153–66.

Williams, A. C. de C., et al., "Psychological Therapies for the Management of Chronic Pain (Excluding Headache) in Adults," *Cochrane Database of Systematic Reviews* 2012, no. 11 (2012): CD007407.

13. Finnerup, N. B., "Nonnarcotic Methods of Pain Management," *New England Journal of Medicine* 380, no. 25 (2019): 2440–48.

Kamper, S. J., et al., "Multidisciplinary Biopsychosocial Rehabilitation for Chronic Low Back Pain: Cochrane Systematic Review and Meta-analysis," *BMJ* 350 (2015).

14. Rosser, B. A., et al., "Online Eye Movement Desensitization and Reprocessing Therapy for Chronic Pain: A Pilot-Controlled Trial," *Journal of EMDR Practice and Research* (2023).

15. Schwartz, A., "EMDR Therapy, Chronic Pain, and Somatic Illness." *Go With That Magazine* 28, no. 1 (2023): 2–11.

16. Ibid.

17. McCracken, L. M., *Contextual Cognitive-Behavioral Therapy for Chronic Pain* (Seattle: IASP Press, 2005).

Dahl, J., and T. Lundgren, *Living Beyond Your Pain: Using Acceptance and Commitment Therapy to Ease Chronic Pain* (Oakland, CA: New Harbinger Publications, 2006).

18. McCracken, L. M., and S. Morley, "The Psychological Flexibility Model: A Basis for Integration and Progress in Psychological Approaches to Chronic Pain Management," *The Journal of Pain* 15, no. 3 (2014): 221–34.

19. Clauw et al., op. cit.

20. Dale and Stacey, op. cit.

21. Andrew et al., op. cit.

22. Patel, K. V., et al., "Prevalence and Impact of Pain Among Older Adults in the United States: Findings from the 2011 National Health and Aging Trends Study," *Pain* 154, no. 12 (2013): 2649–57.

23. Volkow, N. D., and R. Baler, "A Prescription for Better Opioid Prescribing?," *Nature Medicine* 24, no. 10 (2018): 1492–98.

24. Rankin, L., *Sacred Medicine: A Doctor's Quest to Unravel the Mysteries of Healing* (Louisville, KY: Sounds True, 2022).

25. Nørgaard, M. W., "Visualization, a Strategy for Patients to Manage Pain," PhD thesis, Aalborg University, 2018.

26. Ibid.

27. Hilton, L., et al., "Mindfulness Meditation for Chronic Pain: Systematic Review and Meta-analysis," *Annals of Behavioral Medicine* 51, no. 2 (2017): 199–213.

28. Dueñas et al., op. cit.

29. Clauw et al., op. cit.

Geneen, L. J., et al., "Physical Activity and Exercise for Chronic Pain in Adults: An Overview of Cochrane Reviews," *Cochrane Database of Systematic Reviews* 4, no. 4 (2017): CD011279.

30. Snow-Turek, L. A., et al., "Active and Passive Coping Strategies in Chronic Pain Patients," *Pain* 64, no. 3 (1996): 455–462.

31. Finnerup, op. cit.

Jordan, K. P., et al., "Pain That Does Not Interfere with Daily Life—A New Focus for Population Epidemiology and Public Health?," *Pain* 160, no. 2 (2019): 281–85.

32. Snow-Turek et al., op. cit.

33. Edwards, R. R., et al., "The Role of Psychosocial Processes in the Development and Maintenance of Chronic Pain," *The Journal of Pain* 17, no. 9 (2016): T70–92.

Denk, F., et al., "Pain Vulnerability: A Neurobiological Perspective," *Nature Neuroscience* 17, no. 2 (2014): 192–200.

34. Campbell, P., et al., "Prognostic Indicators of Low Back Pain in Primary Care: Five-Year Prospective Study," *The Journal of Pain* 14, no. 8 (2013): 873–83.

35. Picavet, H., et al., "Pain Catastrophizing and Kinesiophobia: Predictors of Chronic Low Back Pain," *American Journal of Epidemiology* 156, no. 11 (2002): 1028–34.

36. Samulowitz, A., et al., "'Brave Men' and 'Emotional Women': A Theory-Guided Literature Review on Gender Bias in Health Care and Gendered Norms Towards Patients with Chronic Pain," *Pain Research and Management* (2018).

37. Ibid.

38. Scott, K. M., et al., "Depression–Anxiety Relationships with Chronic Physical Conditions: Results from the World Mental Health Surveys," *Journal of Affective Disorders* 103, no. 1–3 (2007): 113–20.

21. Sleep

1. American Psychiatric Association, *Diagnostic and Statistical Manual of Mental Disorders, Fifth Edition, Text Revision* (Washington, DC: American Psychiatric Association Publishing, 2022).

2. Ramar, K., et al., "Sleep is Essential to Health: An American Academy of Sleep Medicine Position Statement," *Journal of Clinical Sleep Medicine* 17, no. 10 (2021): 2115–19.

3. Watson, N. F., et al., "Joint Consensus Statement of the American Academy of Sleep Medicine and Sleep Research Society on the Recommended Amount of Sleep for a Healthy Adult: Methodology and Discussion," *Journal of Clinical Sleep Medicine* 38, no. 8 (2015): 931–52.

Luyster, F. S., et al., "Sleep: A Health Imperative," *Sleep* 35, no. 6 (2012): 727–34.

4. Hertenstein, E., et al., "Insomnia as a Predictor of Mental Disorders: A Systematic Review and Meta-analysis," *Sleep Medicine Reviews*, no.43 (2019): 96–105.

5. Williamson, A. A., et al., "Longitudinal sleep problem trajectories are associated with multiple impairments in child well-being," *Journal of Child Psychology and Psychiatry* 61, no. 10 (2020): 1092–103.

6. Walker, M., *Why We Sleep: Unlocking the Power of Sleep and Dreams* (New York: Scribner, 2017).

7. American Psychiatric Association, op. cit.

8. Watson et al., op. cit.

9. Walker, op. cit.

10. American Psychiatric Association, op. cit.

11. Brasure, M., et al., "Psychological and Behavioral Interventions for Managing Insomnia Disorder: An Evidence Report for a Clinical Practice Guideline by the American College of Physicians," *Annals of Internal Medicine* 165, no. 2 (2016): 113–24.

Dopheide, J. A., "Insomnia Overview: Epidemiology, Pathophysiology, Diagnosis and Monitoring, and Nonpharmacologic Therapy," *The American Journal of Managed Care* 26, no. 4 (2020): S76–84.

Qaseem, A.,et al., "Management of Chronic Insomnia Disorder in Adults: A Clinical Practice Guideline from the American College of Physicians," *Annals of Internal Medicine* 165, no. 2 (2016): 125–33.

12. Schutte-Rodin, S., et al., "Clinical Guideline for the Evaluation and Management of Chronic Insomnia in Adults," *Journal of Clinical Sleep Medicine* 4, no. 5 (2008): 487–504.

13. Rios, P., et al., "Comparative Effectiveness and Safety of Pharmacological and Non-Pharmacological Interventions for Insomnia: An Overview of Reviews," *Systematic Reviews* 8, no. 281 (2019).

14. Schutte-Rodin et al., op. cit.

15. MacKenzie, N. E., et al., "Children's Sleep During COVID-19: How Sleep Influences Surviving and Thriving in Families," *Journal of Pediatric Psychology* 46, no. 9 (2021): 1051–62.

16. Ibid.

23. Navigating a Mental Health Crisis

1. "Navigating a Mental Health Crisis," National Alliance on Mental Illness, nami.org/wp-content/uploads/2023/07/Navigating-A-Mental-Health-Crisis.pdf. Accessed May 7, 2024.

2. Ibid.

3. Pistorello, J., et al., "A Randomized Controlled Trial of the Collaborative Assessment and Management of Suicidality (CAMS) Versus Treatment as Usual (TAU) for Suicidal College Students," *Archives of Suicide Research* 25, no. 4 (2021): 765–89.

4. "Mental Health," National Institute of Mental Health, nimh.nih.gov/health/statistics/mental-illness.shtml#part_154910. Accessed May 7, 2024.

5. "Suicide Prevention: Facts About Suicide," Centers for Disease Control and Prevention, cdc.gov/suicide/facts/index.html. Accessed May 7, 2024.

6. "Mental Health by the Numbers," National Alliance on Mental Illness, nami.org/mhstats. Accessed May 7, 2024.

7. Mann, J. J., et al., "Improving Suicide Prevention Through Evidence-Based Strategies: A Systematic Review," *The American Journal of Psychiatry* 178, no. 7 (2021): 611–24.

8. Pattani, A., "Social Media Posts Warn People Not to Call 988. Here's What You Need to Know," NPR, August 25, 2022, npr.org/sections/health-shots/2022/08/11/1116769071/social-media-posts-warn-people-not-to-call-988-heres-what-you-need-to-know.

9. Green, E., and O. Peneff, "An Overview of Police Use of Force Policies and Research," Illinois Criminal Justice Information Authority, August 15, 2022, icjia.illinois.gov/researchhub/articles/an-overview-of-police-use-of-force-policies-and-research.

Crane, L., et al., "Experiences of Autism Spectrum Disorder and Policing in England and Wales: Surveying Police and the Autism Community," *Journal of Autism and Developmental Disorders* 46, no. 6 (2016): 2028–41.

10. Cappellazzo, T. M., "Police Interactions with Mentally Ill Individuals," *The Sociological Imagination: Western's Undergraduate Sociology and Criminology Student Journal* 5, no. 1 (2016): Article 2.

11. Ibid.

12. "Mental Health," op. cit.

"Suicide Prevention: Facts About Suicide," op. cit.

Chatmon, B. N., "Males and Mental Health Stigma," *American Journal of Men's Health* 14, no. 4 (2020).

Eghaneyan, B. H., and E. R. Murphy, "Measuring Mental Illness Stigma Among Hispanics: A Systematic Review," *Stigma and Health* 5, no. 3 (2020): 351–63.

13. "Mental Health, Human Rights and Legislation: Guidance and Practice," World Health Organization and United Nations, iris.who.int/bitstream/han dle/10665/373126/9789240080737-eng. pdf?sequence=1. Accessed May 7, 2024.

14. Ibid.

15. Ibid.

16. "Navigating a Mental Health Crisis," op. cit.

17. Mathias, C. W., et al., "What's the Harm in Asking About Suicidal Ideation?," *Suicide & Life-Threatening Behavior* 42, no. 3 (2012): 341–51.

24. Finding a Mental Health Professional

1. Prusiński, T., "The Strength of Alliance in Individual Psychotherapy and Patient's Wellbeing: The Relationships of the Therapeutic Alliance to Psychological Wellbeing, Satisfaction with Life, and Flourishing in Adult Patients Attending Individual Psychotherapy," *Frontiers in Psychiatry* 13 (2022): 827321.

2. Baier, A. L., et al., "Therapeutic Alliance as a Mediator of Change: A Systematic Review and Evaluation of Research," *Clinical Psychology Review* 82 (2020): 101921.

Fernandez, O. M., et al., "Therapeutic Alliance in the Initial Phase of Psychotherapy with Adolescents: Different Perspectives and Their Association with Therapeutic Outcomes," *Research in Psychotherapy: Psychopathology, Process and Outcome* 19, no. 1 (2016).

3. Lambert, M. J., and D. E. Barley, "Research Summary on the Therapeutic Relationship and Psychotherapy Outcome," *Psychotherapy: Theory, Research, Practice, Training* 38, no. 4 (2001): 357–61.

4. Rogers, C. R., "The Necessary and Sufficient Conditions of Therapeutic Personality Change," *Journal of Consulting Psychology* 21, no. 2 (1957): 95–103.

5. Fernandez, E., et al., "Live Psychotherapy by Video Versus In-Person: A Meta-Analysis of Efficacy and Its Relationship to Types and Targets of Treatment," *Clinical Psychology & Psychotherapy* 28, no. 6 (2021): 1535–49.

25. Navigating Primary Care

1. Thielke, S., et al., "Integrating Mental Health and Primary Care," *Primary Care: Clinics in Office Practice* 34, no. 3 (2007): 571–92.

2. Olfson, M., "The Rise of Primary Care Physicians in the Provision of US Mental Health Care," *Journal of Health Politics, Policy and Law* 41, no. 4 (2016): 559–83.

3. Miller-Matero, L. R., et al., "Integrated Primary Care: Patient Perceptions and the Role of Mental Health Stigma," *Primary Health Care Research & Development* 20 (2019): e48.

4. Asarnow, J. R., et al., "Integrated Medical-Behavioral Care Compared with Usual Primary Care for Child and Adolescent Behavioral Health: A Meta-Analysis," *JAMA Pediatrics* 169, no. 10 (2015): 929–37.

Archer, J., et al., "Collaborative Care for Depression and Anxiety Problems," *Cochrane Database of Systematic Reviews* 10 (2012): CD006525.

Huffman, J. C., et al., "Essential Articles on Collaborative Care Models for the Treatment of Psychiatric Disorders in Medical Settings: A Publication by the Academy of Psychosomatic Medicine Research and Evidence-Based Practice Committee," *Psychosomatics* 55, no. 2 (2014): 109–22.

5. Charles, C., et al., "Shared Decision-Making in the Medical Encounter: What Does It Mean? (or It Takes at Least Two to Tango)," *Social Science & Medicine* 44, no. 5 (1997): 681–92.

6. Hersh, L., et al., "Health Literacy in Primary Care Practice," *American Family Physician* 92, no. 2 (2015): 118–24.

7. Kinchen, E., et al., "Patient and Provider Decision-Making Experiences: A Qualitative Study," *Western Journal of Nursing Research* 43, no. 8 (2021): 713–22.

8. Bodegård, H., et al., "Challenges to Patient Centredness—A Comparison of Patient and Doctor Experiences from Primary Care," *BMC Family Practice* 20, no. 1 (2019): 83.

9. Ibid.

10. Porcerelli, J. H., et al., "Childhood Abuse in Adults in Primary Care: Empirical Findings and Clinical Implications," *International Journal of Psychiatry in Medicine* 52, no. 3 (2017): 265–276. Doi:10.1177/0091217417730290.

11. Kutner, M., et al., "The Health Literacy of America's Adults: Results From the 2003 National Assessment of Adult Literacy," National Center for Education Statistics, 2006.

12. Berkman, N. D., et al., "Low Health Literacy and Health Outcomes: An Updated Systematic Review," *Annals of Internal Medicine* 155, no. 2 (2011): 97–107.

13. Mays, V. M., et al., "Perceived Discrimination in Health Care and Mental Health/Substance Abuse Treatment Among Blacks, Latinos, and Whites," *Medical Care* 55, no. 2 (2017): 173–81.

14. Nair, L., and O. A. Adetayo, "Cultural Competence and Ethnic Diversity in Healthcare," *Plastic and Reconstructive Surgery. Global Open* 7, no. 5 (2019): e2219.

15. Joseph, K. S., et al., "Maternal Mortality in the United States: Recent Trends, Current Status, and Future Considerations," *Obstetrics and Gynecology* 137, no. 5 (2021): 763–71.

16. American Psychiatric Association, *Diagnostic and Statistical Manual of Mental Disorders, Fifth Edition, Text Revision* (Washington, DC: American Psychiatric Association Publishing, 2022).

17. Porter, J., et al., "Revisiting the Time Needed to Provide Adult Primary Care," *Journal of General Internal Medicine* 38, no. 1 (2023): 147–55.

18. "Mental Health in Primary Care: Illusion or Inclusion?," World Health Organization, who.int/docs/default-source/primary-health-care-conference/mental-health.pdf?sfvrsn=8c4621d2_2. Accessed May 7, 2024.

19. Ibid.

26. Navigating Health Insurance and Self-Pay

1. "National Uninsured Rate Reaches an All-Time Low in Early 2023 After Close of ACA Open Enrollment Period," U.S. Department of Health and Human Services, aspe.hhs.gov/sites/default/files/documents/e06a66dfc6f62afc8bb809038dfaebe4/Uninsured-Record-Low-Q12023.pdf. Accessed May 7, 2024.

2. "Access to Care Data 2022," Mental Health America, mhanational.org/issues/2022/mental-health-america-access-care-data. Accessed May 7, 2024.

3. Ibid.

ACKNOWLEDGMENTS

We wish to acknowledge our wonderful clients, from our internships until today, who have taught us so much about strength, resilience, and hope, no matter what obstacles life throws your way. You inspire us every day.

Julie: My immense gratitude and love to my family and friends who comprise some of the kindest, funniest, and most resilient people I know. Mom, Dad, Kiera, and Steve: Don't forget to "wear gloves." Grayson and Nolan, keep being independent and brave. I am thankful to all of the clients, colleagues, and teachers I have had the honor to work alongside and learn from. And to Charity and Nicole, thank you for being wise, generous, and strong women that I am honored to call my friends.

Charity: To my parents who encouraged my love of reading, which grew into a love of writing. Dad, I wish you had gotten to hold this book in your hands; I'm so glad you got to know it was being published. To my siblings, friends, therapists, and colleagues who have taught me through every interaction to be a better person and therapist. To my clients who let me walk alongside them on their journey to heal from trauma. To Severus, Albus, and the chickens for being both great writing companions and distractions. To Julie and Nicole for making this process so much better than I ever thought it could be. And most especially to Tom, for your endless patience and love, bringing me tea while I wrote, being my tech support, listening to all my ideas on our walks, and for teaching me how awesome neurodiversity really is.

Nicole: To all those who trusted me with their stories and vulnerabilities, thank you for granting me the privilege of being witness to your strength, courage, and grace. It is truly the greatest of honors. To my family, thank you for your belief in me. Angelo, thank you for your patience and endless latte refills. Your support is everything. Julie and Charity, I had so much fun on this wild journey with you. You are both brilliant, supportive, and encouraging. Thank you, thank you.

And thank you to our wonderful team at The Experiment Publishing, for believing in this project and helping bring it to life!

INDEX

grief (*continued*)
types of, 129–30
The Grieving Brain
(O'Connor), 129–30
Guided Imagery, 35, 61–62

H

harm reduction, addiction and, 192
harm to self, 78, 93. *See also* Borderline Personality Disorder
health literacy, 251
help, asking for. *See* support, finding
helplines
about, 235
for addiction (Substance Abuse and Mental Health Services Administration), 196
BlackLine (helpline), 17, 235
National Alliance on Mental Illness (NAMI), 17
National Domestic Violence Hotline, 166
National Sexual Assault Hotline, 157
National Suicide and Crisis Lifeline, 17, 119, 228
911, using, 228–30
"warm lines" (peer support hotlines), 228
Helverson, Nicole, 3–4
hunger cues, 180
hyperactivity challenges, 87–88. *See also* Attention-Deficit/Hyperactivity Disorder (ADHD)
hypomanic symptoms, 9–10

I

ice, mammalian dive reflex and, 61
Illness Anxiety Disorder, 252, 267
imaginal exposure, 43
imposter phenomenon (imposter syndrome), 125, 267
impulsivity challenges, 87–88. *See also* Attention-Deficit/ Hyperactivity Disorder (ADHD)
inattention challenges, 87, 88. *See also* Attention-Deficit/ Hyperactivity Disorder (ADHD)
infertility and pregnancy loss, 140–47
abortion rights and, 141

anger about, 140
communicating about, 145
coping difficulty and barriers, 143–45
coping strategies for, 142–43
example of, 146
professional help for, 141–42
reading list and resources for, 147
in-network providers, defined, 259
inpatient therapy/services, defined, 220
insomnia, 9, 208–9. *See also* sleep
insurance and self-pay, navigating, 256–64
barriers to, 261–62
communicating about, 262–63
effective strategies for, 260–61
example, 263
financial issues and paying for therapy, 242–43
paying for therapy and, 242–43, 256
reading list and resources about, 264
self-pay, defined, 259
terminology, 257–60
intake appointments, 239
intensive outpatient program (IOP), defined, 219
intensive therapy, defined, 219
Internal Family Systems Therapy (IFS)
for anxiety, 26
for Borderline Personality Disorder, 80
for chronic pain, 201
defined, 60, 267
for trauma, 69
Interoceptive Exposure, 35, 50
interpersonal relationships, 100–12. *See also* loneliness; social health
barriers to healthy relationships, 105–8
childhood attachment and effect on, 100–1, 102–3
communicating in, 108–10
coping strategies for, 102–5
example, 110–11
loneliness and strengthening of, 114
professional help for, 101
reading list and resources, 111–12
intimate partner violence (IPV), 159–67

communicating about, 164–65
defined, 159–60
escaping from, 161, 162–63
example of, 165–66
National Domestic Violence Hotline, contacting, 166
"power and control wheel," 160
professional help for, 160
reading list and resources for, 167
intrusion, 59
involuntarily committed, defined, 220
"I" statements, 108–9
"Its not logical, it's biological," 150–51

J

job, changing, 122–23. *See also* work stress and burnout
journaling, 23–25, 29, 102, 131, 211
judgment, fear of, 153–54
"just get over it" statements, caution about, 132

K

Ketamine-Assisted Therapy, 80, 228

L

labels, for negative thoughts, 24
Levine, Peter, 268
LGBTQ+
BlackLine (helpline) for, 235
body image and, 173
children, 72
crises and finding support, 230
Developmental Trauma and resources for, 72
institutional exclusion and reproductive justice, 144
sexual assault, 149
licensed clinical social workers, defined, 240
licensed therapists, defined, 240
Linehan, Marsha, 78
loneliness, 113–19
barriers to feeling better, 115–17
communicating about, 117–18
coping strategies for, 114–15
defined, 113–14
example, 118–19

ABOUT THE AUTHORS

JULIE RADICO, PsyD, ABPP, is a board-certified clinical health psychologist with ten years of experience working in primary care settings. In 2023, she opened an independent consulting, coaching, and therapy practice. She earned her doctoral degree in clinical psychology and master's degrees in clinical psychology and counseling as well as clinical health psychology at the Philadelphia College of Osteopathic Medicine.

drjulieradico.com
keep_it_simple_psychology

CHARITY O'REILLY, LPC, is a licensed professional counselor specializing in trauma therapy. She provides intensive trauma therapy for trauma survivors and trains and consults with therapists on trauma-informed practice. She is certified in eye movement desensitization and reprocessing (EMDR) therapy, trauma-focused cognitive behavioral therapy (TF-CBT), and trauma processing yoga.

charityoreilly.com
teawithatraumatherapist

NICOLE HELVERSON, PsyD, is a clinical psychologist in private practice specializing in depression, grief, eating disorders, and anxiety. She also has experience providing therapy in community behavioral health, inpatient psychiatric hospitals, and group practice settings. She attended the Philadelphia College of Osteopathic Medicine, where she earned her doctoral degree in clinical psychology and master's degrees in clinical psychology and counseling as well as clinical health psychology.

drnicolehelverson.com
keep_it_simple_psychology